The Essential Guide for
Patient Safety Officers

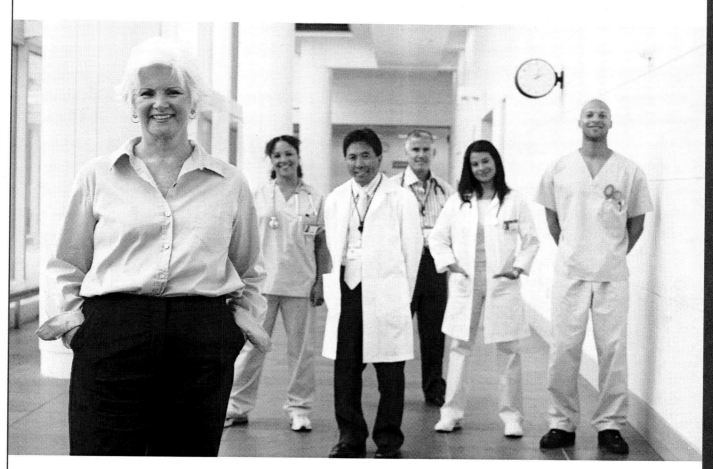

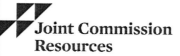

Joint Commission
Resources

Edited by
Allan Frankel, M.D.
Michael Leonard, M.D.
Terri Simmonds, R.N.
Carol Haraden, Ph.D.
with Kathleen B. Vega

Foreword by
Sir Liam Donaldson, M.Sc., M.D.

INSTITUTE FOR
HEALTHCARE
IMPROVEMENT

Executive Editors: Steven Berman and Kristine M. Miller, M.F.A.
Senior Project Manager: Cheryl Firestone
Manager, Publications: Paul Reis
Associate Director, Production: Johanna Harris
Associate Director, Editorial Development: Diane Bell
Executive Director: Catherine Chopp Hinckley, Ph.D.
Vice President, Learning: Charles Macfarlane, F.A.C.H.E.
Reviewers: Donald Kennerly, M.D, Ph.D.; Aileen R. Killen, R.N., Ph.D.; Peter Angood, M.D.; Laura Botwinick; Cathy Hinckley, Ph.D.

Joint Commission Resources Mission

The mission of Joint Commission Resources (JCR) is to continuously improve the safety and quality of health care in the United States and in the international community through the provision of education, publications, consultation, and evaluation services.

Joint Commission Resources educational programs and publications support, but are separate from, the accreditation activities of The Joint Commission. Attendees at Joint Commission Resources educational programs and purchasers of Joint Commission Resources publications receive no special consideration or treatment in, or confidential information about, the accreditation process.

The inclusion of an organization name, product, or service in a Joint Commission publication should not be construed as an endorsement of such organization, product, or service, nor is failure to include an organization name, product, or service to be construed as disapproval.

Joint Commission Resources, Inc. (JCR), a not-for-profit affiliate of The Joint Commission, has been designated by The Joint Commission to publish publications and multimedia products. JCR reproduces and distributes these materials under license from The Joint Commission.

The Institute for Healthcare Improvement (IHI) is an independent not-for-profit organization helping to lead the improvement of health care throughout the world. Founded in 1991 and based in Cambridge, Massachusetts, IHI works to accelerate improvement by building the will for change, cultivating promising concepts for improving patient care, and helping health care systems put those ideas into action.

Printed in the U.S.A. 5 4 3 2 1

Requests for permission to make copies of any part of this work should be mailed to
Permissions Editor
Department of Publications
Joint Commission Resources
One Renaissance Boulevard
Oakbrook Terrace, Illinois 60181
permissions@jcrinc.com

ISBN: 978-1-59940-2345
Library of Congress Control Number: 2008941760

For more information about Joint Commission Resources, please visit http://www.jcrinc.com.

CONTENTS

FOREWORD

Health care is a remarkable industry. Those who work within it are privileged to be in the business of supporting the sick, of reducing suffering, of saving lives. Our care, though, does not always go according to plan. Sometimes it causes suffering; sometimes even death.

The publication of this *Essential Guide* comes at an exciting time for the rapidly evolving field of patient safety. Just a decade ago, the issue of patient safety had barely entered our collective consciousness. Scattered throughout health care systems were smatterings of insight that mistakes were occurring—repeatedly, in some instances—and that avoidable errors were killing and harming some of the patients in our care. There was, however, little to connect the pieces of the jigsaw—no systematised approach to understanding errors and learning from them, no common language to facilitate this, and little appreciation of the fundamental shifts in the very culture of health care that would be vital to tackling the problems of medical error.

At the turn of the millennium, the inescapable reality dawned. The Institute of Medicine's landmark report *To Err is Human*[1] estimated the number of people dying in the United States because of medical error to be equivalent to a jumbo jet crash on every single day of the year. There was a clear moral imperative to act—rapidly, decisively, and effectively.

The will to act soon became apparent at the highest levels. In 2002, the World Health Assembly passed a resolution to form the World Alliance for Patient Safety, a global body that I have chaired since its inception. Through our First Global Patient Safety Challenge, ministers of countries representing more than 80% of the world's population have pledged to address one of the great global issues—that of health care–associated infections.

Yet I have seen the immense challenges of translating will into action. Directives from the top do not automatically result in change—far from it. Rather, real improvement occurs through the efforts of individuals within hospitals and other health care institutions. Such individuals must have not just the drive but also the insight, knowledge, and tools necessary to adapt their organizations' systems, processes, and culture to reduce the occurrence of error. Such expertise has evolved over the last decade, through extensive study and collaboration within the health care industry and beyond.

The Institute for Healthcare Improvement has developed a world-leading expertise in the multifaceted domains required to tackle the challenges of improving patient safety. Their intensive training program for patient safety officers has allowed attendees to benefit from the firsthand knowledge, skills, and experience of international experts in the field. I am pleased that Joint Commission Resources, which has provided so much guidance to health care organizations on the improvement of quality and patient safety, has teamed with the program's faculty to develop this hands-on guide.

Within this book, you will read how the patient safety field has adopted approaches used successfully by other industries; appreciating how these can be applied synergistically is fascinating. The aviation industry has provided a number of useful tools for examining errors and understanding their causation. It has also given us the valuable concept of Crew Resource Management. Inspiration for increasing efficiency has come, in particular, from the "Lean" production system pioneered by Toyota.

I am delighted that this book gives such emphasis to the creation of a "safety culture." This is perhaps the greatest challenge for every organization: to infuse a culture of safety throughout an organization, to create an organization in which safety is not a project, a target or an initiative, but at the core of its very being; to enthuse every colleague, from the front line to the boardroom—this is the great, yet vital, challenge that faces the patient safety officer. Sometimes terms such as "culture" and "communication" are sprinkled throughout high-level documents. Specific tools, processes, and pathways are far more concrete and manageable concepts. The patient safety field is, out of necessity, developing an expertise in how truly to engage with organizational culture and how to translate the broad objective of patient safety into concrete aims that can be tackled using specific approaches. Whatever the temptation to disregard safety culture, I would recommend that you pay particularly close attention to this area.

I have personally seen the immense value of involving patients and their families in the process of understanding and reducing error, and am delighted that this approach is promoted within this book. I vividly remember one father, whose daughter died following misdiagnosis of a serious illness, saying to me, "Patient safety is my life now." Inviting such individuals to be involved as you improve safety within your organization is emotionally challenging, but they can provide a key perspective, are highly motivated to help, and ensure that everybody in your organization is acutely aware of the importance of what you are doing.

The relationship between technology and patient safety is particularly interesting. This book rightly describes technology as a double-edged sword. Electronic systems such as computerized physician order entry systems have tremendous potential to help eliminate errors, but they are not a short cut. They require sensible introduction, monitoring, and an active safety culture to achieve their full potential. An understanding of how humans interact and "work around" technology is vital. While technology has tremendous potential to improve safety, examples in this book demonstrate that its misuse—because of poor training, maintenance, or introduction— has significant potential to introduce harm.

The maxim *primum non nocere*—first, do no harm— has been attributed to various leading thinkers in health care through the ages, from Hippocrates in the 4th century BC to Florence Nightingale in the 19th century. In 1859 Nightingale reflected, "It may seem a strange principle to enunciate as the very first requirement in a hospital that it should do the sick no harm." The principle may seem obvious, but translating it into reality requires vision and it requires skill. The challenge to every reader of this book is to engage their organization in closing the gap between intention and effective implementation. If you are able to apply the collective expertise and wisdom in this book, the health care industry might be on the way to rendering the need to repeatedly express Florence Nightingale's maxim, "first, do no harm," truly redundant.

Your challenge is to make real our collective vision of patient safety being at the heart of how we think and work, deep in the very fabric of our organizations, at the core of all of our systems. Patient safety should not ultimately be a field in itself but be deeply engrained throughout the health care industry. I wish you well.

Sir Liam Donaldson
Chief Medical Officer, England
Chair, World Alliance for Patient Safety

REFERENCE

1. Institute of Medicine: *To Err Is Human: Building a Safer Health System.* Washington, DC National Academy Press, 2000.

CONTRIBUTORS

EDITORS/AUTHORS

Allan Frankel, M.D.
Faculty, Institute for Healthcare Improvement
Principal, Lotus Forum
allan.frankel@lotusforum.com

Michael Leonard, M.D.
Physician Leader for Patient Safety, Kaiser Permanente
Faculty, Institute for Healthcare Improvement
Principal, Pascal Metrics
michael.leonard@pascalmetrics.com

Terri Simmonds, R.N.
Principal, Safe & Reliable Healthcare
Faculty and Director, Institute for Healthcare Improvement
terri.c.simmonds@gmail.com

Carol Haraden, Ph.D.
Vice President, Institute for Healthcare Improvement
charaden@ihi.org

Kathleen B. Vega
Writer
kvega@mindspring.com

AUTHORS

Mary Ann Abrams, M.D., M.P.H.
Clinical Performance Improvement, Iowa Health System
abramsma@ihs.org

Asif Ahmad, M.B.A., M.S.
Vice President, Diagnostic Services and Chief Information
    Officer, Duke University Health System
asif.ahmad@duke.edu

Barbara Balik, R.N., Ed.D.
Faculty, Institute for Healthcare Improvement
Consultant, Pascal Metrics
barbara.balik@pascalmetrics.com

Doug Bonacum, M.B.A.
Vice President for Safety, Kaiser Permanente
doug.bonacum@kp.org

Maureen Connor, R.N., M.P.H.
Vice President for Quality Improvement and Risk Management,
    Dana-Farber Cancer Institute
maureen_connor@dfci.harvard.edu

Frank Federico, Pharm.D.
Executive Director for Strategic Partners, Institute for Healthcare
    Improvement
ffederico@ihi.org

Michael Fox, R.N., B.S.N.
Perinatal Director, Pascal Metrics
perinatal@consultant.com

Karen Frush, R.N., M.D.
Chief Patient Safety Officer, Duke University Health System
Vice Chair of Strategic Initiatives, Department of Pediatrics,
    Duke University Medical Center
frush002@mc.duke.edu

Christen Fullwood
Research Coordinator, Johns Hopkins University Quality and
    Safety Research Group
cfullwo1@jhmi.edu

Sarah Grillo, M.H.A.
Director of Operations, Pascal Metrics
sarah.grillo@pascalmetrics.com

Annie Herlik, R.N., J.D.
Director of National Risk Management, Kaiser Permanente
annie.herlik@kp.org

Andrew P. Knight, M.A., M.S., A.B.D.
Director of Research & Development, Pascal Metrics
Doctoral Candidate, The Wharton School, University of
    Pennsylvania
andrew.knight@pascalmetrics.com

Robert Lloyd, Ph.D.
Executive Director of Performance Improvement, Institute for
    Healthcare Improvement
rlloyd@ihi.org

David Munch, M.D.
Chief Clinical and Quality Officer, Exempla Lutheran Medical
    Center
munchd@exempla.org

Gail Nielsen
Clinical Performance Improvement, Iowa Health
Faculty, Institute for Healthcare Improvement
nielsega@ihs.org

Peter J. Pronovost, M.D., Ph.D.
Director, Johns Hopkins University Quality and Safety Research
    Group
ppronovo@jhmi.edu

Roger Resar, M.D.
Senior Fellow, Institute for Healthcare Improvement
rresar@ihi.org

William Rupp, M.D.
CEO, Mayo Health System
rupp.william@mayo.edu

J. Bryan Sexton, Ph.D., M.A.
Director of Safety Culture Research and Practice, Johns Hopkins
    University Quality and Safety Research Group
bryan.sexton@opensafety.org

Introduction

CREATING A ROAD MAP FOR PATIENT SAFETY

Allan Frankel, Michael Leonard, Terri Simmonds, **and** *Carol Haraden*

Anna Rodriguez—a 27-year-old mother of young twins— enters a preeminent teaching hospital for arthroscopic knee surgery on a Tuesday morning after a holiday weekend. The surgery department has a full schedule with both elective and emergency surgeries scheduled.

Ms. Rodriguez is prepped in the preoperative area by Eileen Page, a registered nurse and 20-year veteran of the hospital. Per the organization's protocol, Ms. Rodriguez is supposed to receive prophylactic antibiotics one hour before her surgery. Because it is approaching 45 minutes before Ms. Rodriguez's scheduled surgical start time, Ms. Page is in a hurry to give the preoperative antibiotics. Busy with another patient as well, Ms. Page has dozens of procedural steps she must perform to ready both patients for surgery, and she inadvertently overlooks checking the medical record for allergies. Unfortunately, Ms. Rodriguez is allergic to certain antibiotics, including the ones that Ms. Page is about to administer. Buried in the many pages of the medical record is a note about a significant systemic reaction to antibiotics, but no one has noted Ms. Rodriguez's allergies in a prominent place where Ms. Page could easily be reminded.

Because she is in a hurry, Ms. Page tries quickly to explain to Ms. Rodriguez what she is doing. Ms. Rodriguez is from Venezuela and does not speak English well. Ms. Page does not speak Spanish, so communication is sketchy at best. The Spanish-speaking nurse on staff is busy attending to another patient, and Ms. Page is trying to move Ms. Rodriguez quickly into surgery so the surgery schedule will not be too adversely impacted. Organization leadership has repeatedly stressed to frontline staff the importance of adhering to the surgery schedule—cases must start on time. In fact, management closely tracks the percentage of cases that start on time and continually pushes to improve it.

As Ms. Page begins to administer the antibiotics, Ms. Rodriguez becomes agitated because of her lack of ability to communicate clearly. Although Ms. Page notices the agitation, she assumes Ms. Rodriguez is just nervous before her surgery.

Approximately 45 minutes after receiving the antibiotics, Ms. Rodriguez is brought into the operating room (OR). The surgeon is anxious to get started and very curtly calls the OR team together to begin surgery. As the surgery begins, the OR staff notices that Ms. Rodriguez's vital signs are quite abnormal, and she appears to be in respiratory distress. The team is unclear as to what is happening, and the surgeon barks out an order to one of the circulating nurses to quickly check the medical record for any clues. The OR team tries to stabilize Ms. Rodriguez, but she suffers cardiovascular collapse, is ultimately resuscitated, but suffers significant severe neurologic injury.

After quickly reviewing the medical record, the team realizes the nature of the problem. Ms. Page is devastated. The media swarms onto the campus of the medical center, asking many difficult questions that the leaders of the institution are unable to answer to their satisfaction. Ms. Rodriguez's family is kept in the dark about what really happened to their loved one, so they retain an attorney to represent them. The public is outraged by this tragic mistake and start demanding that the hospital do something to prevent this kind of event in the future. Leadership in the organization begins to look for someone to blame for the incident, and Ms. Page seems like a good candidate.

Eventually, hospital leadership goes before the press and public and commit to eliminating medical errors in their facility and improving safety. They hire a consultant, launch some safety initiatives that target medication errors, and feel confident their work is making a difference. However, the root causes of the event that occurred in the OR are still present in the organization: lack of communication, lack of teamwork, lack of patient involvement, lack of reliable processes, lack of organizational emphasis on safety and reliability, and the inability of the organization to continuously learn from its mistakes. While the implemented safety initiatives may improve medication safety in the organization for a short time, they serve only as a Band-Aid for a deeper, more long-term problem.

What if this operating room scenario or one like it occurred in your organization? Would the response have been the same? Does your organization and its senior leadership value and commit to a culture of safety? Reliable systems? Teamwork and communication? Is the accountability system in your organization structured to protect the hardworking nurse like Ms. Page, who inadvertently makes a mistake because of a series of system errors? Or is it designed to identify fault and place blame? When errors do occur, does your organization have a systematic approach to responding and learning from them? Does your organization have an open and honest disclosure process? Are patients involved in their care? Do they have a voice within the organization? If your answers to any of these questions are "no," you are not alone. However, you are also nowhere near where you need to be in providing safe and reliable health care.

ALL WORK AND NOT ENOUGH GAIN

Since the Institute of Medicine's 1999 landmark report on medical error,[1] many health care organizations have focused on reducing medical errors and enhancing the safety of patients. Despite this focus, the number of medical errors occurring in the United States has not appreciably changed. While intentions are good, there is often a substantial gap between the safe and reliable care we know to be effective and the current care that is provided. As a whole, health care organizations are still experiencing error at an unacceptable rate and are continuing to harm people in repetitive and predictable ways.

While there have been some very successful individual efforts to address the issue of safety, much of the work has been fragmented or focused on specific small areas. These efforts have shown some short-term success, but long-term improvement has remained elusive. The creation of patient safety officers within health care is an important step on this journey.

ADDRESSING THE ROOT OF THE PROBLEM

The primary reason for the lack of progress is that organizations are not addressing the roots of the safety problem. Yes, decreasing error is important, but it cannot happen without an environment that supports a systematic approach to creating and maintaining reliable processes and continuous learning. In other words, before an organization can realize sustained improvement, it must commit to designing reliable processes that prevent or mitigate the effects of human error and establish a culture where teamwork thrives, people talk about mistakes, and everyone is committed to learning and improvement. Once an organization achieves an environment of reliability and continuous learning, then patient safety becomes a property or characteristic of the organization and, by definition, the organization starts to reduce errors.

MAKING SAFETY AN ORGANIZATIONWIDE IMPERATIVE

So how do you achieve an environment where reliable processes exist and continuous learning is an intrinsic value? It doesn't happen by just telling employees to try harder to be safe. It requires a systematic approach that addresses the fundamental ways in which providers interact and provide care. Such a systematic approach involves four critical components[2]:

1. A strategy, which focuses on reliability and continuous learning. This strategy represents an organization's basic values and vision as well as its goals.

2. A structure, which consistently supports the strategy and helps integrate it into the accepted way of doing business. Such a structure builds the appropriate framework, designates the appropriate resources, and defines the reporting relationships that effectively support the strategy.

3. An environment or culture that supports the structure and ensures the proper execution of deliverable outcomes to meet strategic objectives, such as reduced error and enhanced patient safety.

4. Clear outcomes and associated metrics that are visible, both internally to the people doing the work and externally to the market and the public. These outcomes and metrics help drive consistent improvement within the organization.

The Essential Guide for Patient Safety Officers provides a road map for organizations to create the necessary strategy, structure, environment, and metrics that focus on reliability and improve patient safety. Based on the Institute for Healthcare Improvement's Patient Safety Officer Course—a synthesis of patient safety experts' collective experience—each brief, easy-to-digest chapter focuses on a different stop along the map, as follows:

- The Role of Leadership
- Safety Culture
- Accountability
- Reliability and Resilience
- Systemic Flow of Information
- Teamwork and Communication
- Direct Observation and Feedback
- Disclosure
- Patient Involvement
- Technology
- Measurement Strategies
- Process Improvement Methods
- Effective Implementation Strategies

Despite the specificity of its title, this book is designed to help anyone in an organization improve the safety of care provided to patients from the patient safety officer to front-line staff who are charged with and/or interested in improving the provision of care. Even if your organization does not have a patient safety officer per se, you can benefit from this publication as it discusses the critical steps involved in enhancing patient safety throughout an organization and ensuring the reliability of care. By the time you finish reading this book, you should have a clear understanding of what is involved in creating and sustaining a culture of safe and reliable care. You will be armed with tips and tools to apply to your own organization and examples from other organizations that have engaged in these efforts.

The concepts discussed within this book may be simple in theory, but they can be quite challenging to implement without complete organizational support of a strategic approach to improvement. It takes a commitment from all levels to systematically drive this work and achieve success. However, by incorporating the different elements discussed in this book into everyday work, organizations can take a step toward reliability, learn from mistakes, and continuously improve, enhance, and achieve patient safety. It is important to note that while the overall goal of safe and reliable care may seem somewhat daunting, there is a great deal of low-hanging fruit, and committed individuals can and do make a huge difference in how we care for patients.

REFERENCES

1. Kohn L., et al.: *To Err Is Human: Building a Safer Health System.* Washington, DC: Institute of Medicine of the National Acadamies, Nov. 1, 1999.
2. Frankel A.S., Leonard M.W., Denham C.R.: Fair and just culture, team behavior, and leadership engagement: The tools to achieve high reliability. *Health Serv Res* 41:1690–1709, 2006.

ACKNOWLEDGMENTS

The editors first and foremost acknowledge Kathleen B. Vega, without whose patience, persistence, and writing expertise this book would not have been possible. To our colleagues who continue to teach us and advance our understanding of safe care delivery, we are certainly in your debt. As for individuals, Steve Berman, Don Berwick, Richard Bohmer, Jeff Brown, Penny Carver, James Conway, Donald Kennerly, Aileen Killen, David Lawrence, Lucian Leape, Tami Merryman, Kristine Miller, Paul Preston, Paul Reis, Jane Roessner, Paul Uhlig, and John Whittington deserve special mention.

This book is dedicated to those who have taught us about the critical importance of safe care, and particularly those who paid far too dear a price.

Chapter One

THE ROLE OF LEADERSHIP

William Rupp, Doug Bonacum, Karen Frush, Barbara Balik, and *Carol Haraden*

The most important factor in achieving safe patient care is overt, palpable, and continuous commitment from organization leadership to create a strategy, establish a structure, and foster an environment that encourages, supports, and requires safe and reliable care. Such a strategy, structure, and environment cannot exist without the commitment of leadership—senior leaders, boards of directors, and physician and nursing leadership—and cannot be realized by simply a grass roots approach. Performance improvement and enhanced safety may occur in small areas but improvement cannot be sustained or expanded throughout the organization.

Partnering with formal and informal leaders, especially senior executives, to achieve safer care is an essential part of a patient safety officer's role. This chapter will assist you and your leadership partners in achieving safer care outcomes.

As discussed in the Introduction, achieving safety is not a one-time or short-term effort. Major progress requires a multifaceted leadership approach,[1] implemented and revisited over time, and includes activities such as assessing a culture for safety,[2] responding to data, striving for high reliability,[3] requiring transparency,[4] fostering communication and teamwork,[5,6] setting meaningful goals,[7] and sharing outcomes.

The following are seven essential leadership steps to take to achieve health care safety:

1. Assess the culture for safety and act to close the gaps.
2. Understand the science of improvement and reliability—strive to be a high reliability organization.
3. Foster transparency.
4. Create a leadership promise.
5. Engage physicians and nurses, especially those in executive and formal leadership roles.
6. Hire for what you aspire to become.
7. Involve board members in the safety journey.

ASSESS THE CULTURE FOR SAFETY AND ACT TO CLOSE THE GAPS

Creating a culture based on safety typically requires a cultural shift in the way caregivers, medical staff, patients, and leadership view the health care organization and their respective roles in it. To be successful, organization leadership must encourage, support, and drive change from the common and inaccurate belief that a health care organization is a collection of smart, hard-working individuals trying really hard to provide safe care to the evidence-based view that a health care organization is a complex set of teams of professionals, patients, families, and leaders who work together to systematically provide the most effective care in the most efficient way.

One of the first steps in changing a culture involves assessing the culture in its current form. As discussed further in Chapter 2, cultural assessment involves looking at a variety of data—both quantitative and qualitative—that measure culture, including staff perceptions of safety, teamwork, management, stress recognition, and job satisfaction.

Other data can also reveal information about your organization's culture, including reports or lack of reports about potential safety issues that come into a spontaneous reporting system, analyses or lack of analyses of near misses, and stories of concerns from caregivers gleaned during Executive WalkRounds™ and/or direct observation in care settings.[8] While all these activities are discussed further in later chapters, they are mentioned here to reinforce the point that leaders must commit to using a variety of types and sources of data to learn about an organization, its culture, its strengths, and its weaknesses. Leaders must be open to seeing problems while consistently looking and listening for issues that may exist beyond a leader's attention. Avoiding the temptation to judge problems as rarities is difficult but very important.

Effectively interacting with data involves not only analyzing and responding to them, but also considerable effort in ensuring that the most useful data are collected. It is important to note that more data are not necessarily better and can just get you lost in the analytic process; the key is to select focused, actionable data.

The clearer your organization can be on what data will be most relevant to assess the organization's culture and determine areas of improvement the better.

UNDERSTAND THE SCIENCE OF IMPROVEMENT AND RELIABILITY

Health care is a complex endeavor. The processes of health care can and should be designed to anticipate and mitigate human error, ensure that processes occur the way they are designed, and achieve the outcomes they need to achieve. In other words, processes must be designed so they are reliable. As discussed in Chapter 4, designing reliable processes that mitigate human error involves critical assessment of current processes, careful planning, and the use of the science of reliability. Leaders must learn that the science of reliability is essential to their role. They must understand and accept the science behind this work and teach others—including physicians—about it. Most health care leaders and professionals did not learn the science of reliability in their professional education, thus it is likely they may not even know it exists. It is the responsibility of leadership to understand and apply that science to the daily work of the organization.

STRIVE TO BE A HIGH-RELIABILITY ORGANIZATION

While reliable processes are one component of a reliable organization, there are other aspects involved in embedding reliability at the cultural level, an activity that is essential to working toward functioning as a high-reliability organization (HRO).

At their most basic level, HROs experience fewer accidents despite typically operating in "risky" and complex environments.[9] Examples of HROs include the aviation, hazardous chemicals, and aeronautical industries. Such industries achieve reliability because they actively seek to know what they don't know, design systems to make available important knowledge that relates to a problem to everyone in the organization, learn in a quick and efficient manner, aggressively avoid organizational arrogance or the belief "errors cannot happen here," train organization staff to recognize and respond to system abnormalities, empower staff to act, and design redundant systems to catch problems early.[10] In other words, an HRO expects its organization and its subsystems, regardless of how reliably they are designed, to fail, and the HRO works very hard to avoid known sources of failure while preparing for unexpected failures, so that the organization can minimize both the frequency and impact of future failures.[3]

Those looking to migrate their organizations toward HRO status should begin by clarifying the leadership role involved, committing to regularly assessing stories that provide a window to understand the organization's culture—reviewed annually—and implementing a set of expected behaviors, activities, and initiatives that other organizations have used to successfully drive change. Many of these behaviors, activities, and initiatives are described throughout this book. (*See* Case Study 1-1 on page 8.)

FOSTER TRANSPARENCY

Transparency in health care involves openness in communication, acknowledging error, offering an apology when harm occurs, defining accountability at all levels in the organization, and committing to system improvement. A transparent organization does not try to hide mistakes, but acknowledges that errors occur and works to fix the systems that ultimately cause those errors. Such an organization accepts that it is not perfect, and continuously works to identify areas of improvement.

A culture is transparent only if its leaders define, role model, and cultivate that transparency. There are many ways to do this, including the following:

• Openly discuss failure. Talk about, discuss, and analyze issues, errors, and risks with frontline staff, medical staff, patients, families, and the public.

• Share data—both good and bad—on performance with frontline staff, medical staff, patients, families, and the public.

• Provide avenues for feedback. This includes Executive WalkRounds™,[11] glitch books, spontaneous reporting systems, surveys, complaint hotlines, and so forth. (*See* Chapter 5 for a further discussion of these feedback mechanisms.)

• Respond to that feedback both with communication and improvement in a timely manner to encourage further feedback.

• Develop leadership skills across the organization for transparency, so the ability to consistently share data, safely learn from failures, and reinforce an accountability model is a foundational organizational property at all levels.

• Be consistent when responding to medical errors. Leaders should establish an accountability system to differentiate between system errors and individual errors and apply that system consistently across the organization.[12,13] (*See* Chapter 3 for a further discussion of accountability.)

Though the following points are not directly related to transparency, active work in these areas is important in supporting a transparent culture:

• Foster teamwork and effective communication across the organization. (*See* Chapter 6 for a further discussion of teamwork and communication.)

• Involve and develop the capacity of all stakeholders in improvement, including frontline staff, medical staff, patients, and families.[14,15]

• Involve patients in their care through multidisciplinary rounds, transition reports, and eliminating visiting restrictions; talk openly and honestly with patients and families when things go wrong; apologize; and assure ongoing support for patients and families who have been harmed.[16] (*See* Chapters 8 and 9 for more information.)

Many organizations are fearful of transparency as they believe it will reveal flaws and increase lawsuits. The concern is that if the organization exposes its weaknesses, people will capitalize on those weaknesses to the detriment of the organization. However, there is research that shows that this is not what typically happens. In fact, being transparent often increases trust with patients and families. When one hospital in the Pacific Northwest was open and honest about a high-profile medical error, the public responded positively to the organization, believing that the organization was working to provide the most appropriate care and, when it failed, was open and honest about it. When Paul Levy, the CEO of Beth Israel Deaconess Medical Center located in Boston, openly discussed a wrong site surgery error on his weekly blog, it stirred a spirited discussion within the medical community,[17] but also resulted in appreciation from the public that he was open, honest, and transparent.

Being transparent also has the benefit of improving employee morale and engagement in improvement efforts. Sharing data about strengths and weaknesses excites and motvates staff to participate in improvement efforts. It

reflects a commitment to be candid and continually improve.

Sharing Outcomes Is Part of Transparency

When implementing new initiatives, it is critical to share the results and show if a process does, in fact, improve patient outcomes and increase efficiency. To sustain physician and staff involvement in improvement, they must believe that improvement is being realized and the process does work. For example, if your organization is implementing a new insulin protocol, you need to have graphs everywhere showing the reduction in episodes of hyper- and hypoglycemia. This allows the physicians, nurses, and other staff to see that "Hey, this really does work." Measure and display the results on important things—show them that together, you're actually making things better.

CREATE A LEADERSHIP PROMISE

One specific action that organization leaders can do to help verbalize their commitment to transparency and high reliability is to create a Leadership Promise. This is a document that clearly delineates the role of the leader in safety, reliability, and performance improvement. Figure 1-1 on page 5 is an example of one organization's leadership promise.

ENGAGE PHYSICIANS

A critical leadership group that must be engaged in your organization's safety efforts is physicians. Without the support, participation, and enthusiasm of physicians, safety improvement efforts will have trouble getting off the ground. Physicians have a huge impact on the quality of care delivered, clinical variation, and resource consumption. Effective physician relationships with nursing leadership, frontline nurses, pharmacists, and other caregivers are essential for the consistent delivery of safe, high-quality care. Therefore, any changes in the way care is designed and delivered require physician acceptance and participation, either as individuals or as a professional body.[18]

Engaging physicians in improvement initiatives has historically been a challenge for health care organizations, because physicians' primary professional and business focus is their own practice—the quality of care they personally deliver and the economics associated with that care. In many instances, the priorities for physicians seem out of alignment with the quality issues faced by the larger health care system in which they work. At best, physicians have little time to spare for the organization's quality agenda. At worst, relationships become strained because the physicians' quality and business agendas appear to be in conflict with those of the health care organization.[18]

The way physicians are trained also contributes to difficulties in engaging them. The physician culture is largely based on personal responsibility for patient outcomes and contributes to physicians' fierce attachment to individual autonomy. This cultural element puts physicians in conflict with a systematic approach to patient care and also leads naturally to a blaming culture. Physicians are taught that "If we work and study hard enough, we won't make a mistake." This leads them to believe that if a mistake does happen, it is their—or others'—fault. They often fail to see their role in a larger system, the many components of which came together to form a risky situation that resulted in error and potential harm.

Compounding this cultural bias is the fact that most physicians rarely experience the negative consequences of a medical error. There are approximately 700,000 physicians in the United States, and roughly 50,000–100,000 fatal medical errors each year. Doing the math, that nets down to a physician being involved in a serious or fatal medical error a couple of times over the course of his or her career. From a physician's perspective, this hardly seems like an epidemic. What physicians fail to realize is that their patients' good clinical outcomes are not solely a result of their talents as physicians, but also of the effectiveness of the systems in which physicians use those talents.

Despite the many potential difficulties in engaging physicians, it is critical to do so if performance improvement efforts are going to succeed. So how can organizations engage physicians? One effective way is to match organizational performance improvement goals with the quality goals physicians value. What is most important to physicians? Patients. Physicians care a lot about patient outcomes because they care about their patients and want to make sure that the care provided to patients is appropriate and effective. In addition, physicians believe that patient outcomes reflect on their reputations. In their minds, a patient who has successful surgery credits the surgeon and not the system that supports the surgeon.

Whether right or wrong, physicians often do not consider their reputations related to the health care organization and therefore do not value the improvement efforts targeted to improving organization quality, such as efforts focused on reducing length of stay or increasing patient throughput. These improvements are often described in regulatory or business terms rather than linking with physicians' professional or personal motivations. This framing of the language often fails to capture the heart of physicians. Physicians care about initiatives that affect their patients' health outcomes, such as fewer infections, lower mortality, and other indicators of outstanding care. Even enhancing patient satisfaction is important to physicians only if the satisfaction being enhanced relates directly to their patients.

In addition to improved patient outcomes, physicians value their time. For most physicians, time is a rare commodity. They are juggling multiple patients with complicated conditions and need to make decisions in a time frame that is at best short. Physicians will embrace anything that improves efficiency and saves time. Processes that result in less wasted time, fewer hassles, reduced bottlenecks and delays, and minimized rework will gain their support. In some cases, the importance of time can trump the importance of patient outcomes. In other words, if an effort improves outcomes but costs more time, physicians most likely will be unable to do it.

If organization leadership can show physicians that new processes are making patient outcomes better and giving the physicians more time, then physicians will be more likely to support performance improvement efforts, thus enhancing the probability that such efforts will be successful.

It's important to note that by mirroring organizational performance improvement objectives with that of physicians, your organization does not have to sacrifice its own quality goals. For example, if you pursue better patient outcomes and increased physician time, you decrease length of stay, enhance efficiency, and improve financial performance. In other words, organizational outcomes will improve as a by-product of patient outcomes and time efficiency.

Some practical considerations in involving physicians:
• Physician quality has historically been associated with peer review, which is generally perceived as a punitive process, not an opportunity to learn. Reframing the conversation as an opportunity to improve the quality of care provided is essential. Teaching about system error and having a model of accountability is key to supporting this cultural shift.

Figure 1-1. Not on My Watch

Following is one organization's Leadership Promise. It is a written document that organizations can use to help verbalize a leader's commitment to safety and reliability.

I am at the helm of a medical center that intends on providing the safest hospital care in the United States by the end of the year [fill in year]. We will do this by eliminating all preventable death and injury to our patients as we continue to pursue a workplace free of injury to our staff. In partnership with our physician and union leaders, our safety aim is routinely communicated to every employee and physician, and more recently, to our patients.

I actively oversee a 3-year plan to achieve our goal that builds off of the great work we've already begun. By actively oversee, I mean that I receive monthly progress reports and require corrective action plans to close identified gaps. In concert with this activity, I personally track a small number of hospitalwide patient safety measures that are routinely updated and made fully transparent to our staff and to our members; these measures include hospital risk adjusted mortality, a global harm rate generated by use of the IHI Global Trigger Tool, bundle compliance for bloodstream and surgical site infections as well as ventilator-associated pneumonia (VAP), and never events.

I have tied our patient safety aim to other hospitalwide initiatives, including improving flow, eliminating workplace injuries to our staff, and improving service. In the process, my CFO has become a true patient safety champion, realizing that safe, reliable care is no accident, and no accident is good for our bottom line. In addition, each member of my senior leadership team is required to cosponsor a patient safety improvement initiative. This helps them better understand the complexity of providing safe, reliable care, and allows them to better connect their activities to our aim.

Each week, I personally spend about four hours on matters directly related to the provision of safe, reliable care. During this time, I:

✔ Conduct Executive WalkRounds™ and review reports indicating the status of issues that staff have identified during our time together

✔ Review all significant events and sign off on each one with a statement that says I have reviewed the case and that it appears the corrective action plan will significantly reduce the risk of recurrence. . .of course, I'm not the only one who makes this certification, but I am the last one. I also make sure that lessons learned from both our own, and other medical centers' events, are shared with our frontline practitioners. After all, they are the ones who have a need to know.

✔ Spend 10 minutes at new employee and physician orientation to make clear, in no uncertain terms, my views of patient safety and my expectations of them. I also let them know that my door is always open to safety and how they can contact me.

✔ Follow up on reports of unsafe practitioners and make sure that we are not only addressing identified issues of competency, but identifying issues related to collaboration, respect, and organizational values.

✔ Visit with our member-driven, patient safety advisory council and hear directly from our members what's concerning them and what's going well.

✔ Act as an executive sponsor of improvement initiatives related to eliminating unwarranted variation in workflow and process. . .medicine is complex enough without having eight different ways of doing the same thing.

✔ Review resource requests concerning patient safety that have been denied at lower levels in the organization. I agree with most of the decisions made, but want everyone to understand, the buck stops here with respect to patient safety.

✔ Visit with one of our performance improvement teams on the floor to hear and see specifically how their work is going. We currently have initiatives related to eliminating preventable infection, medication, and birth-related injuries. They are all on 90- to 120-day performance improvement cycles and so I see remarkable progress every week.

By far, the hardest thing I do is to meet with patients/families who have suffered a significant, preventable injury while in our care. It may also be the most meaningful thing I do.

On an annual basis, I ensure that the current state of the organization's patient safety culture is measured. In between, I am driving the creation of a just culture by demanding a brief on every patient safety–related event where part of our response strategy has been to use discipline. I'm all for accountability. . .and to ensuring that our response is "Just."

As more and more patient safety demands are placed on the organization by state, federal, and accrediting bodies, I sponsor a review of our staffing and structure to ensure that we have the resources in place to do what's needed. I periodically update my own knowledge of patient safety and demand my executive team does the same. This year, five members of our team are attending the IHI Annual Forum.

As well as I think we generally do here, I recognize that to go from where we are to where we want to be is going to require a relentless commitment on my part to improve patient safety. Only I can productively direct efforts to foster the culture and commitment required to address the underlying systems causes of medical error and harm.

Preventable Death and Injury? Not on My Watch. . .Not in My Region. . .Not in My Organization!

Source: Doug Bonacum. Used with permission.

- Physicians love to give opinions—create a physician advisory group to do patient safety work.

- Be willing to strategically pay physicians four to eight hours a month to be "Patient Safety Champions." Paying less than they would earn often works; what is critical is to acknowledge, their time is valuable.

- Don't waste their time. Physicians are very action oriented—they want to see results.

- Working on risk-adjusted mortality is a great subject; physicians are interested in this.

- Physicians respond to clinical data more than opinion. Measure and obtain hard data and survey data that will withstand scrutiny. When the data lose credibility, recovering it is very difficult. Measure items that are important to physicians; ask them, don't assume.

- Consistently reinforce the message that effective teamwork is critically important for delivering safe, high-quality care.

- In debates and with disagreement, always focus on what's best for patients. That helps anchor the conversation around a common goal.

Following the 80/20 Rule

When trying to engage physicians, it is difficult to work with every physician in the hospital and ensure their comprehensive support and involvement. In all likelihood, 80% of your organization's medical staff rarely steps foot in the hospital. These are not the individuals on whom you should initially focus your efforts. It is the 20% of staff members who spend the majority of their time working in the hospital—the hospitalists, residents, full-time staff, and medical staff members who regularly practice in the hospital—who have a clear, vested interest in improving clinical care.

Within that 20%, you should identify those individuals who embrace change and value performance improvement. These champions can help colead initiatives, address issues, and generate support and engagement of others. These early leaders need skills training, such as training in performance improvement and conflict resolution; support to learn from others, including time to network with others, go to conferences, and do site visits; and effective partners to achieve outcomes, such as a successful nurse coleader. When the 20% are on board, the remaining critical mass of practitioners will learn from their experiences and even add to the initial improvement work.

Make Physicians Partners, Not Customers

Along with aligning priorities with physicians, leaders must work to shift the physician's perspective on his or her role in the organization. Many hospital leaders believe that physicians are important customers who make care decisions while the organization leadership runs the finances and facilities. Likewise, physicians often believe they must have complete autonomy for everything and take personal responsibility only for the patients they take care of directly.

These viewpoints are not productive for the organization, physicians, or patients. To provide the most effective and safe care, patients should be the only customers of a health care organization, and physicians should be partners in providing care to those customers. Physician perspective must shift from being responsible only for their patients to being responsible for the systems that take care of all the patients in the hospital; and leaders must make physicians accountable to improve those systems rather than remaining bystanders.

Organizational leadership must set expectations for this perspective shift and support those expectations by consistent practice. Leaders should work with physicians who understand that the patient is the only customer and want to build systems together to support patient needs. Most physicians went into medicine because they want to provide care for people and thus should support the idea of putting the patient at the center of the work.

Unfortunately, some physicians may not like this perspective shift, and in those cases leaders must respond consistently. Physicians who are not willing to give up autonomy for a systematic approach should be encouraged to practice elsewhere. Consider the following scenario.

At the quarterly meeting of the Board Quality Committee, a community board member asks about the medical record delinquency data. The Medical Director says "Yes, we have one or two serial offenders, but one of them is our key trauma surgeon. His op notes and D/C summaries are always months behind. But if we suspended his privileges, as called for in the bylaws, our trauma program would pretty much shut down."

In your institution, what would happen next? Ideally, the trauma surgeon should be held accountable to the same standards as everyone else and disciplined accordingly if he is not willing to change his behavior. If you do not have a single standard—one set of rules—it is very hard to preserve accountability and have a culture that is perceived as fair. This is a key point.

ENGAGE NURSES

Organizations that are going to be successful need to invest in a skilled, stable nursing workforce. A simple measure of stability is your organization's annual rate of voluntary nursing turnover. Ideally, it should be close to zero, such as the 0.4% rate at the Dana-Farber Cancer Institute in Boston.[19] With national averages ranging around 10%, where is your organization?[20]

The current cost to replace a nurse in America is about $50,000.[21] Paying large sums of money to trade down—replace skilled people with other options—makes no sense. Estimates are that we will be approximately 500,000 nurses short in the United States by 2020.[22,23] We now do things we never used to do, such as putting brand new graduates in intensive care units, operating rooms, and other high-acuity areas without a few years to develop expertise. Having skilled people at the bedside is essential for safe care and organizational health.

What are the keys to a healthy nursing environment?

• Valuing and rewarding an environment that requires and attracts better educated nurses, acknowledges their value, and supports ongoing learning

• Creating a nursing leadership structure that provides skilled nurse leaders and managers to support frontline nurses

• Fostering collegial nurse-physician relationships

• Building and sustaining a culture in which nurses, and all employees, are treated with respect[24]

• Committing to programs that help build organizational excellence in nursing, such as the American Association of Critical Care Nurses Health Work Environments Standard, magnet status, and so forth

All of these responsibilities fall directly within the purview of senior leaders.

HIRE FOR WHAT YOU ASPIRE TO BECOME

While the military has proven through processes like boot camp, that it is possible to rapidly shape another's attitudes and behaviors in alignment with an organization's aspirations, successful companies like Southwest Airlines have found it equally effective to hire the right people in the first place. If your hiring and credentialing process isn't grounded in finding and selecting candidates—physicians, nurses, other clinicians, support staff—who possess a desire to serve,

good communication skills, an eagerness to work in teams, a commitment to excellence, and an appreciation for feedback, becoming a reliable and safe organization will take much longer and be much harder than it otherwise should. While orientation, ongoing training, and daily reinforcement of safety values are essential ingredients in going from good to great in this area, why not give yourself a head start and get the right people on the bus to begin with?[25]

INVOLVE BOARD LEADERSHIP IN SAFETY

Physicians and nurses aren't the only groups that are critical to patient safety efforts. Another crucial stakeholder is your organization's board of directors. According to Donald Berwick, president and CEO of the Institute for Healthcare Improvement (IHI), "Historically, boards have assumed that they are responsible for the fiscal integrity, reputation, and lay management of the hospital, but that responsibility for care lies with the clinical staff, not with the board. For many boards, medical care, itself, is remarkably foreign terrain. Yet, in a time of increasing corporate accountability, consumer voice, and system complexity, this view will no longer suffice, if it ever did. A large share of the accountability for the safety and quality of care rests firmly in the boardroom. . . . Cultural changes that support patient safety require leadership and in the final analysis, defining the organization's strategic intent and priorities is the responsibility of those who govern the organization."[26]

As Berwick implies, the first step in involving the board in safety and quality efforts is the simple recognition that it is the board's duty in the first place.[26] Better patient outcomes are associated with boards that do the following:

• The board spends more than 25% of its time on quality issues.

• The board receives a formal quality performance measurement report.

• There is a high level of interaction between the board and the medical staff on quality strategy.

• The senior executives' compensation is based in part on quality improvement (QI) performance.

• The CEO is identified as the person with the greatest impact on QI.[27]

According to IHI, to assume a major leadership role in improving clinical quality and reducing harm, there are six things all boards should do[26]:

1. Set aims. Set a specific aim to reduce harm this year.

Case Study 1-1. Cincinnati Children's Hospital Medical Center (CCHMC)

One organization that has taken the safety and reliability message to heart is Cincinnati Children's Hospital Medical Center (CCHMC), a 475-bed, nationally recognized pediatric treatment and research center in Cincinnati, Ohio. In 2005 the CCHMC board of trustees targeted 18 areas for improvement, from surgical site infections to asthma care to moving patients efficiently through the system, applying 99 specific measures to track progress. "While the moral case was clear," says board chairman Lee Carter, "it was also a business decision. You get what you measure and what you pay for, so we're measuring and paying for improvement." Indeed, the year-end bonuses of CCHMC senior managers, once based only on meeting financial goals, are now 70% dependent on meeting stipulated quality improvement goals.

Board involvement didn't end there, says Carter. "There's a saying—'the currency of leadership is attention'—and this board pays a lot of attention." The patient care committee, which Carter leads, meets once a month for presentations by improvement teams throughout the hospital. "If a team isn't moving as well toward its goals as they would like, we work on figuring out what can be done and how the board can help. If they're moving even better than expected, we discuss whether the goal should be reset. For us, progress reports aren't just words and numbers on a page; they're living documents."

Carter acknowledges that achieving some of CCHMC's goals may take quite awhile. "We want to improve long-term functionality outcomes for chronic conditions such as cystic fibrosis, but it's not easy work and you don't know where the tipping point is. You have to just keep going without necessarily seeing an end in sight."

Transparency and "absolute alignment" between the board and senior staff is the key to moving forward, says Carter. "We won't adjust our expectations to make people look better or feel better but, at the same time, we're all working together. Everyone is on the same side." In fact, says Carter, more than half of the quality improvement component in senior management bonuses is based on general improvement throughout the hospital; less than a third is based on improvement within a manager's own area of responsibility. "If someone is having a hard time, everyone's first instinct is to say, 'What can I do to help you?'" Just as gratifying, though, says Carter, is the pride generated by successful teamwork. "When I lead a tour in the hospital, I see good statistics posted on the walls, even in the bathrooms. Our people are just so motivated by what they've been able to accomplish."

One example is CCHMC's progress on reducing ventilator-associated pneumonia (VAP), which can develop when an intensive care patient on a breathing tube accidentally aspirates fluid or bacteria. "We went from delivering perfect care for children with six common conditions 80% of the time to delivering it 95% of the time," says Uma Kotagal, M.B.B.S., M.Sc., director of CCHMC's Health Policy and Clinical Effectiveness division. "We then applied what we learned to VAP, where in three to four months we were delivering all components of the VAP bundle close to 100% of the time."

Lee Carter is pleased but not entirely surprised by results like this. "We planted a flag," he says. "This is what happens when you're very, very focused."[28,29]

Make an explicit, public commitment to measurable quality improvement—such as reducing unnecessary mortality and harm—establishing a clear aim for the facility or system.

2. Get data and hear stories. Select and review progress toward safer care as the first agenda item at every board meeting, grounded in transparency, and putting a "human face" on harm data.

3. Establish and monitor system-level measures. Identify a small group of organizationwide "roll-up" measures of patient safety, such as facilitywide harm or risk-adjusted mortality. Update the measures continually and make them transparent to the entire organization and all of its customers.

4. Change the environment, policies, and culture. Commit to establishing and maintaining an environment that is respectful, fair, and just for all who experience the

pain and loss as a result of avoidable harm and adverse outcomes—the patients, their families, and the staff at the sharp end of error.

5. Learn . . . starting with the board. Develop your capability as a board. Learn about how "best in the world" boards work with executive and physician leaders to reduce harm. Set an expectation for similar levels of education and training for all staff.

6. Establish executive accountability. Oversee the effective execution of a plan to achieve your aim to reduce harm, including executive team accountability for clear quality improvement targets.

In addition to IHI's perspective on involving boards in quality and safety efforts, The Joint Commission emphasizes the importance of organization leaders communicating about safety and quality. Through its Leadership standards,

The Joint Commission requires organization leaders—including members of the governing body, senior managers, and leaders of the organized medical staff—to communicate with each other on a regular basis with respect to issues of safety and quality.

Getting this level of leadership may be challenging, but in its absence, change will be difficult to effect and even more difficult to sustain. Consider beginning the process by engaging each leadership group (the board of directors, CEO, and physician and nursing leaders) in a conversation regarding their level of awareness of the issues, how they view their accountability in this arena, whether they think the organization has the capacity for change, and what explicit actions might be taken to close performance gaps. Consider creating a program in which every new board member and senior leader needs to spend two to four hours shadowing a frontline caregiver. This is a critical perspective they all need. Consider having a patient safety–focused retreat for senior leaders with outside speakers. Often it is easier for external experts to deliver the message of quality and safety and push for significant commitment and improvement.

In an article related to this topic,[30] Denham et al. states: "Awareness is the first critical dimension. . . . Leaders must be aware of performance gaps before they can commit. . . Accountability of leaders for closing performance gaps is critical . . . leaders need to be directly and personally accountable to close the performance gaps . . . [However, leaders] will fail to close [performance gaps] if their organizations do not have the ability to adopt new practices and technologies. The dimension of ability may be measured as capacity. It includes investment in knowledge, skills, compensated staff time, and 'dark green dollars.'"

To determine if your organization leadership is ready to be effective in achieving safety, initially assess board and senior team performance; and work with the CEO to develop his or her own Leadership Promise using the one provided earlier in this chapter as a guide. Finally, evaluate whether you have respected physicians and other leaders who are or are willing to act as champions of change. They must be willing to publicly commit their support among their peers and express the importance of various efforts. They must also be willing to openly deal with resistance from their colleagues in a constructive manner and insist on a professional culture that won't tolerate nonprofessional behavior.[31] Clear board and CEO support and commitment on these last two points is critically important for success.

In summary, committed, capable and engaged leadership is essential to systematically improving care and building a culture that makes it sustainable.

REFERENCES

1. Bennis W.G., Thomas R.J.: *Leading for a Lifetime.* Boston: Harvard Business School Press, 2007.
2. Rose J., et al.: A leadership framework for culture change in health care. *Jt Comm J Qual Patient Saf* 32:433–442, Aug. 2006.
3. Weick K., Sutcliffe K.: Managing the unexpected. San Francisco: Jossey-Bass, 2001.
4. Connor M., et al.: Creating a fair and just culture: One institution's path toward organizational change. *Jt Comm J Qual Patient Saf* 33:617–624, Oct. 2007.
5. Nunes J., McFerran S.: The perinatal patient safety project: New can be great. *Permanente Journal* 9:25–27, Winter 2005.
6. Leonard M., Graham S., Bonacum D.: The human factor: The critical importance of effective teamwork and communication in providing safe care. *Qual Saf Health Care* 13(suppl. 1):i85–i90, 2004.
7. Pryor D., et al.: The clinical transformation of Ascension health: Eliminating all preventable injuries and death. *Jt Comm J Qual Patient Saf* 32:299–308, Jun. 2006.
8. Mazzocco K., et al.: Surgical team behaviors and patient outcomes. *Am J Surg* Sep. 11, 2008.
9. Frankel A., Haraden C.: Shuttling toward a safety culture: Healthcare can learn from probe panel's findings on the Columbia disaster. *Mod Healthc* 34:21, Jan. 2004.
10. Roberts K.H., Bea R.G.: "Must accidents happen: Lessons from high reliability organizations." *Acade Manage Exec* pp. 70–79, Aug. 2001.
11. Frankel A., Grillo S.P., Baker E.G., et al.: Patient safety leadership WalkRounds™ at Partners Healthcare: Learning from implementation. *Jt Comm J Qual Patient Saf* 31:423–437, 2005.
12. Reason J.: Managing the Risks of Organizational Accidents. Brookfield, VT: Ashgate, 1997.
13. Outcome Engineering, LLC: The Just Culture Community. Home page: http://www.justculture.org (accessed Nov. 10, 2008).
14. University of Pittsburgh Medical Center: *Condition H.* http://www.upmc.com/aboutupmc/qualityinnovation/centerforquality improvementandinnovation/pages/conditionh.aspx (accessed Nov. 10, 2008).
15. Institute for Family Centered Care. Home page: http://www.family centeredcare.org (accessed Nov. 10, 2008).
16. Adult Patient & Family Advisory Council. Dana Farber Cancer Institute. http://www.dana-farber.org/pat/pfac/adult-advisory/default.html (accessed Nov. 10, 2008).
17. Beth Israel Deaconess Medical Center: *Chat with Paul Levy.* http://www.bidmc.harvard.edu/YourHealth/BIDMCInteractive/Chats/2008/November/ChatwithPaulLevy.aspx (accessed Nov. 10, 2008).
18. Reinertsen J., et al.: Engaging physicians in a shared quality approach. Institute for Healthcare Improvement: Innovation Series, 2007.
19. Hayes C., et al.: Retaining Oncology Nurses: Strategies for Today's Nurse Leaders. Oncology Nursing Forum. http://www.ons.org/publications/journals/ONF/Volume32/Issue6/32061087.asp (accessed Nov. 10, 2008).
20. DeFontes J., Surbida S.: Preoperative safety briefing project. *Permanente Journal* 8:21–27, Spring 2004.
21. Jones C.B., Gates M.: The costs and benefits of nurse turnover: A business case for nurse retention. *The Online J Issues Nurs* 12(3), 2007.
22. Buerhaus P., et al.: Implications of an aging registered nurse workforce. *JAMA* 283:2948–2954, 2000.

23. Buerhaus P., et al.: *The Future of the Nursing Workforce in the United States: Data, Trends and Implications*, Jones and Bartlett Publishers. http://www.jbpub.com/catalog/9780763756840 (accessed Nov. 17, 2008).

24. Edmondson A.C.: Managing the risk of learning: Psychological safety in work teams. *International Handbook of Organizational Teamwork*. London: Blackwell, 2002.

25. Collins J.: *Good to Great: Why Some Companies Make the Leap—And Others Don't*. London: Random House Business Books, 2001.

26. *Institute for Healthcare Improvement: The Power of Having the Board on Board*. http://www.ihi.org/IHI/Topics/LeadingSystemImprovement/Leadership/ImprovementStories/FSThePowerofHavingtheBoardonBoard.htm (accessed Nov. 10, 2008).

27. Vaughn T., et al.: Engagement of leadership in quality improvement initiatives: Executive quality improvement survey results. *J Patient Safety* 2:2–9, 2006.

28. Britto M.T., et al.: Cincinnati Children's Hospital Medical Center: Transforming care for children and families. *Jt Comm J Qual Patient Saf* 32:541–548, Oct. 2006.

29. National Association of Children's Hospitals and Related Institutions: Pursuing perfection: Transforming children's healthcare.
http://www.childrenshospitals.net/AM/Template.cfm?Section=Homepage&CONTENTID=14165&TEMPLATE=/CM/ContentDisplay.cfm (accessed Jan. 6, 2009).

30. Frankel A.S., Leonard M.W., Denham C.R.: Fair and just culture, team behavior, and leadership engagement: The tools to achieve high reliability. *Health Serv Res* 41:1690–1709, 2006.

Chapter Two

ASSESSING AND IMPROVING SAFETY CULTURE

J. Bryan Sexton, Sarah Grillo, Christen Fullwood, **and** *Peter J. Pronovost*

The practical definition of safety culture is "the way we do things around here." That is, the norms, practices, values, and beliefs of the people working in a given nursing unit or clinical area. Ultimately, it is the local context and environment in which care is delivered.

Safety culture is not a one-dimensional concept, but has multiple dimensions. Some concepts that make up a safety culture include the following:

- Perceptions of teamwork (including norms of speaking up about problems)
- Perceptions of norms and behaviors related to patient safety and quality of care. This is sometimes known as safety climate. (*See* Sidebar 2-1 on page 12.)
- Job satisfaction
- Perceptions of management (at the clinical area and hospital levels)
- Stress recognition. This is the acknowledgement of how performance is influenced by stressors, such as lack of sleep, production pressures, or disruptive behaviors.
- Adequacy of training and supervision
- Institutional learning and responses to error
- Adequacy and availability of equipment, information, and processes
- Reporting infrastructure
- Feedback and communication
- Beliefs about causes of errors and adverse events

A clinical area may be very strong in some dimensions—such as the ability to collaborate with colleagues—but weak in others—such as having an understanding of the relationship between stress and error. For example, almost 40% of clinical areas with a very good teamwork climate also have low stress recognition scores, meaning that they are good at the "how" of communication but lack some of the

"what," which is knowing where and when problems are going to surface.

Overall, a clinical area with a strong safety culture demonstrates effective coordination of care, sees mistakes as opportunities to learn, and has engaged caregivers who proactively and thoughtfully bring solutions forward to their nurse manager/unit director. Conversely, a weak safety culture is one in which caregivers don't communicate, managers respond to mistakes by blaming and training, and caregivers either fail to use existing safety infrastructures or use them as opportunities to complain and vent their frustrations.

Safety culture is a relatively stable phenomenon in a given clinical area if left alone, but it is also quite responsive to interventions and events, such as introducing new technology to a unit, changes in medical or nursing leadership, greater use of agency staff, or changes in geographic location (for example, a new building). These are just some of the events that introduce disruption into a clinical area and can bring down safety culture scores.

It is becoming increasingly clear that safety culture affects the quality of care provided in a clinical area. Research has shown that clinical areas with a strong safety culture have more satisfied patients and staff. A weak safety culture correlates with several of the following red flags for patient harm:

- Decubitus ulcers in medical/surgical units
- Delays in operating room and intensive care unit (ICU)
- Bloodstream infections in the ICU
- Ventilator-associated pneumonia in the ICU
- Wrong-site surgeries
- Postoperative sepsis

- Postoperative infections
- Nursing turnover
- Absenteeism
- Low incident reporting rates
- Staff burnout

ASSESSING SAFETY CULTURE

So how do you know if you, your clinical area, your department, or your organization has a strong safety culture? The best way is to measure it. Assessing a safety culture is important for the following reasons:

- To get baseline data prior to an intervention that might affect culture
- To get a multidimensional profile of the cultural strengths and weaknesses within a clinical area
- To assist in selecting an intervention that is most appropriate for improving quality and safety in a specific context
- To allow quality, safety, and risk leadership to prioritize which clinical areas across the hospital need help, and which do not
- For clinical areas that are struggling, to diagnose specific issues that need to be addressed (for example "The conflicts in this clinical area are not resolved appropriately, and this is pulling down the teamwork climate overall.")
- To use grass-roots efforts of establishing the consensus views in a clinical area to build awareness about the importance of patient safety, teamwork, and quality improvement opportunities
- To drive improvement by establishing a baseline, making the data-driven case for change, and remeasuring at 12–18 month intervals to track changes in patient safety over time

Assessing safety culture allows hospitals and clinical areas to "see themselves" and gain insight into relationships that people often don't feel safe discussing openly. It depersonalizes the conversation, to make it about norms and empirical data, rather than "he said/she said" anecdotes surfaced by strong personalities at a meeting with limited attendance.

Some leaders may believe that such a process is not necessary as they "understand" their culture and its limitations. However, health care executives are typically more optimistic than frontline staff about the strength of the organization's safety culture and the effectiveness of teamwork or patient

---

Sidebar 2-1. The Difference Between Safety Climate and Safety Culture

The lines between these two concepts are becoming increasingly blurred, but the academic distinction between the two remains. Safety culture is measured by anthropologists and ethnographers who look at the history, artifacts, symbols, and infrastructure to assess a construct that is deeper and more stable than climate. Alternatively, constructs such as teamwork climate, or safety climate are more of a snapshot of the broader culture in a clinical area at a given moment in time, so they are more closely related to clinical and operational outcomes, and more responsive to interventions. Metaphorically, culture is like a vast and complex set of interconnected highway systems, while climate is the traffic that darts about on the surface. Simply said, climate is measured with survey questions like "I would feel safe being treated here as a patient," and is more actionable and responsive than the deeper construct of culture.

Outside of health care, safety climate research has received much attention over the past two decades, including within railways[1], nuclear power plants[2], commercial aviation[3], manufacturing[4,5], industrial facilities,[6,7] construction,[8] road administration[9], and restaurants[10]. In high-reliability industries, such as commercial aviation, petrochemical platforms, and nuclear power plants, safety climate is used as a proactive metric of safety to compliment traditional retrospective metrics such as fatalities, incidents, and accidents.

Safety climate scores predict unsafe behaviors,[11,12] injury rates,[4,10] safety-specific organizational citizenship behaviors,[13] and accidents.[7,11]

Despite the large and growing body of research in other high-risk work settings, safety climate research in health care is still in the early stages. Early evidence indicates that safety climate is linked to clinical and operational outcomes,[14–16] and is improvable.[14,15,17,18]

---

safety norms in a given clinical area. In fact, in the absence of incoming data streams, executives tend to overestimate the quality of teamwork and patient safety relative to frontline staff by a large margin, with views that are twice to four times as positive!

Focus on the Clinical Area Level Versus Organizationwide Assessments

Culture, like politics, is local. The culture in your organization's ICU could be strong and robust, but 20 feet down the hall, the medical/surgical unit is a miserable place to be.

A frontline nurse in Unit X doesn't really care what the *hospital* culture is, so much as how his or her actions are going to be viewed within the context of his or her specific *unit* and that specific situation. So while looking at a hospital-wide measurement of safety culture is interesting, it is more important to study the norms in a given clinical area. In addition, there is more variability between units within a typical hospital than there is between hospitals. Because interventions to improve safety are implemented at the clinical area level, it is critical to understand culture at that level. Indeed, there is a great deal of variability between clinical areas, as Figures 2-1 and 2-2 (right) demonstrate.

When assessing safety culture, it is important to perform the assessment across an entire hospital or system while capturing the information and tracking response rates at the clinical area level. This lets you look at the strengths and weaknesses within the institution, but also identify clinical areas that are doing very well and those that are doing poorly. By listening to frontline assessments you may focus your efforts, your executives' attention, and your patient safety resources on the clinical areas that need help. (*See* Figures 2-3 and 2-4 on pages 14 and 15.)

First, target those clinical areas reporting a lack of consensus that the culture is healthy—for example, any clinical area in which less than 60% of respondents report good safety norms and behaviors (safety climate). Conversely, clinical areas in which 60% or more report a good safety climate generally feel comfortable talking about patient harm, have physician champions, are already filling out incident reports, and don't need as much structure and facilitation.

TOOLS FOR MEASURING SAFETY CULTURE

To effectively assess safety culture it is helpful to use a systematic approach involving a validated instrument that meets a variety of theoretical and statistical tests. In response to national interest, including The Joint Commission's 2009 Leadership standards calling for routine culture measurement using a valid instrument at the clinical area level, the number of instruments an organization can use to measure safety culture has grown. The selection and use of a safety culture survey instrument has become an important strategic decision for hospital leaders. Following is a brief discussion of the two tools that are most widely used, and

Figure 2-1. Safety Climate in Michigan

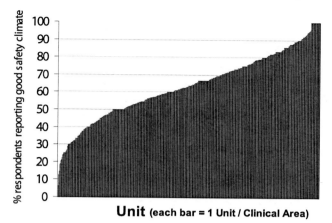

The statewide response rate in Michigan in 2007 was 73%, with 23,789 completed surveys from 48 hospitals.

Source: Bryan Sexton. Used with permission.

Figure 2-2. Safety Climate Across Johns Hopkins Hospital

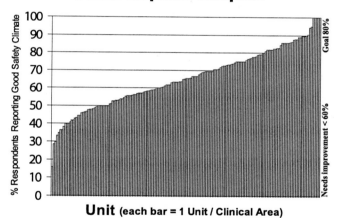

The housewide response rate for Johns Hopkins Hospital in 2007 was 75%, with 4,798 completed surveys across 163 clinical areas.

Source: Bryan Sexton. Used with permission.

how they work.

Safety Attitudes Questionnaire

The Safety Attitudes Questionnaire (SAQ) was developed by one of the authors of this chapter [JBS] over the course of 10 years of validation and reliability research and is a valid instrument for capturing frontline caregiver assess-

Figure 2-3. Safety Culture Varies More by Clinical Area Than by Hospital

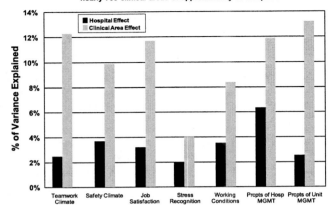

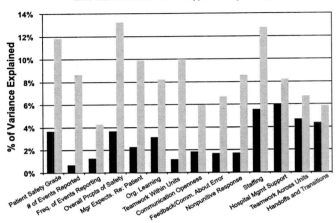

These figures demonstrate variability at the hospital level relative to the clinical area level using the Safety Attitudes Questionnaire and the AHRQ Hospital Survey on Patient Safety Culture. Variance decompositions were conducted using nearly 15,000 SAQ responses from more than 700 clinical areas of approximately 50 hospitals, and nearly 14,000 AHRQ responses from more than 300 clinical areas of approximately 25 hospitals.

Source: Bryan Sexton. Used with permission.

ments of themes such as teamwork, patient safety, trust in management, and so forth. Survey items within the questionnaire were determined based on attitudinal surveys in aviation, observations of caregivers at work, focus groups with caregivers, a review of the literature, and roundtable discussions with subject-matter experts.

The SAQ survey is widely used and accepted in more than 2,000 hospitals in the United States and abroad, with translations available in 12 languages. The SAQ is also widely used in patient safety and quality improvement research, where it has been coupled with improvement concepts, such as briefings, daily goals, Comprehensive Unit-Based Safety Programs (CUSP), and Executive WalkRounds™, with demonstrated impact on culture, patient outcomes, and the fiscal bottom line. To date, the SAQ domain scores—such as teamwork climate and safety climate—have been linked to annual nurse turnover, blood stream infections, ventilator-associated pneumonia, and a variety of other clinical and operational outcomes.

The widely used SAQ Short Form can be used in any inpatient or outpatient clinical area across a hospital or health care system. The survey is one side of one page, with 30 questions divided into the following six different scales:

1. Teamwork climate
2. Job satisfaction
3. Perceptions of management (at the clinical area and hospital level)
4. Safety climate
5. Working conditions
6. Stress recognition

In addition, the survey has demographic questions requesting information such as job position, gender, years experience, and whether one's specialty is primarily adult, pediatrics, or both. Respondents answer questions using a five-point Likert Scale (disagree strongly, disagree slightly, neutral, agree slightly, agree strongly), and "not applicable" is also an option. The survey takes approximately five to seven minutes to complete. After respondents complete the survey using a specific technique that garners high response rates[19], the climate scores and detailed results are generated using published processes for calculating[20] and for feeding back[21] results to frontline staff in a way that is diagnostic and actionable.

With statewide and nationwide administrations of the SAQ recurring every year, there is a large and growing archive of thousands of hospitals for benchmarking purposes.

Figure 2-4. Teamwork Climate in Michigan

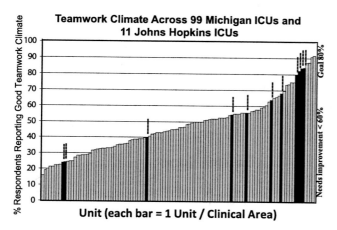

Teamwork Climate Across 99 Michigan ICUs and 11 Johns Hopkins ICUs

Teamwork Climate varies across 99 ICUs in one state (REF 31), from 16% to 92% of the caregivers reporting good teamwork in their unit. Moreover, the dark bars indicate 11 Johns Hopkins ICUs, and illustrate that even within one type of clinical area (ICU) within one institution; there is tremendous variability across clinical areas.

Source: Bryan Sexton. Used with permission.

Agency for Healthcare Research and Quality's Hospital Survey on Patient Safety Culture[22]

This is a publicly available tool that helps organizations conduct a hospitalwide safety assessment. Like the SAQ, the Hospital Survey on Patient Safety Culture can be completed by any hospital staff member, but it is best suited for the following individuals:

• Hospital staff who have direct contact or interaction with patients (clinical staff, such as nurses, or nonclinical staff, such as unit clerks)

• Hospital staff who may not have direct contact or interaction with patients but whose work directly affects patient care (staff in units such as pharmacy, laboratory/pathology)

• Hospital-employed physicians who spend most of their work hours in the hospital (emergency department physicians, hospitalists, pathologists)

• Hospital supervisors, managers, and administrators

There are a total of 51 items in the survey, and it takes approximately 10 minutes to complete. Most of the items use Agree/Disagree or Never/Always response categories to anchor the scales. There is room for written comments at the

end of the survey.

The survey places an emphasis on patient safety issues and error and event reporting. It measures seven unit-level aspects of safety culture:

1. Supervisor/manager expectations and actions promoting safety
2. Organizational learning/continuous improvement
3. Teamwork within units
4. Communication openness
5. Feedback and communication about error
6. Nonpunitive response to error
7. Staffing

In addition, the survey measures three hospital-level aspects of safety culture:

1. Hospital management support for patient safety
2. Teamwork across hospital units
3. Hospital handoffs and transitions

Finally, four perceived outcome variables are included:

1. Overall perceptions of safety
2. Frequency of event reporting
3. Patient safety grade (of the hospital unit)
4. Number of events reported

To help organizations benchmark their survey results against other hospitals, the Agency for Healthcare Research and Quality (AHRQ) established the Hospital Survey on Patient Safety Culture Comparative Database as a central repository for data. Since 2006, hundreds of U.S. hospitals that administered the AHRQ survey have voluntarily submitted their data for inclusion in the database.

Hospitals wanting to compare their hospital's patient safety culture survey results to those of other hospitals can use the comparative results in the 2008 Comparative Database Report to benchmark a culture of patient safety in their institutions.

Using the Hospital Survey on Patient Safety Culture as a starting point, new surveys addressing resident safety culture in nursing homes and patient safety culture in ambulatory outpatient medical offices are under development. Each of the new surveys will contain new and revised items assessing dimensions that more accurately apply to each setting. (The SAQ has already been validated for use in ambulatory and medical office building settings.[23])

How to Select and Effectively Utilize a Survey Instrument

When choosing a survey instrument, keep the following points in mind:

• Versatility. In the absence of a gold standard for patient safety, a safety culture survey needs to be versatile enough to be used across clinical areas and caregiver types. The more the survey instrument is targeted to appeal to the way a busy and/or tired clinician thinks, the more acceptance it will have, and the higher response rates will be. Clinicians are quick to say "You must be talking about somebody else," so using a versatile instrument is critical.

• Psychometric validity. Within the survey, performance of items should stand up over time and correlate well with what's being surveyed. The survey needs to be validated using traditional statistical techniques as well as the latest methods of multilevel modeling and use of inter-class correlations and indexes of consensus within a set of respondents. Optimally, the survey has been developed and refined in an academic environment with attention to both scientific rigor and the practical needs of leaders and unit managers. Surveys that are psychometrically valid, but difficult to interpret or use by nurse managers, are as useless as surveys that are psychometrically inadequate.

• Predictive validity. Ideally, an organization should be able to correlate survey results with operational and clinical outcomes, such as blood stream infection rates, annual nurse turnover rates, delays in initiating care, and so forth.

• Ease of use. There are options that range from conducting a survey entirely in-house, without using any external resources, to conducting a survey that relies exclusively on external experts to help collect, manage, and analyze feedback and to maintain the dataset over time. What is important to remember is that someone, somewhere, must do the work of tracking response rates, cleaning up datasets, generating reports, feeding them back to front-line staff, and tracking the impact of interventions on culture in specific clinical areas over time. To assume that any safety culture survey is without cost would be a mistake, as the efforts of quality and safety managers, analysts, and unit managers to interpret and feed back results in a productive way must be taken into account. Organizations may want to talk to their counterparts in other hospitals to see what their experiences have been with different instruments.

• Benchmarking capability. Tools that can be used, for example, to benchmark one ICU against a statewide distribution of other ICUs, or a national sample of 100 ICUs, strongly appeal to nurse managers and unit directors. This "apples to apples" comparison is as important as the "apples to oranges" comparison of the ICU relative to all of the other clinical areas in the same hospital. So the quality of the benchmarking dataset is critical, meaning the methods used to collect and aggregate the data from different sites must be consistent, and the sites allowed into the benchmarking dataset must have high response rates and be representative of the larger population.

It is important to choose carefully when selecting an instrument, as it will be repeatedly used over time. Switching versions of surveys can be challenging if there are some clinical areas that have trend data with good response rates, while others consistently fail to garner adequate response rates.

IMPLEMENTING THE SURVEY

As you begin to implement a safety culture assessment survey, consider the following points:

• How will you administer the survey? Although the survey can be administered in a variety of ways, the most popular method is to give it to a large group during the first 10 minutes of a staff meeting, in-service, or other educational training session. The captive audience with protected time in the room facilitates high response with little coordination. Other methods of administration include hand delivery (often for physicians), mailing the survey, or providing it online. Electronic administrations require widespread access to the Internet and have traditionally resulted in low response rates and require someone to monitor implementation and actively work to get a significant response.

Response rates are important because with low response rates the data lose validity, diagnosticity, and actionability. To obtain reliable data, you should strive for 80% response, but approximately 60% is the minimum needed. Survey studies with less than 60% response rates are not even accepted for consideration at top-tier medical journals. Low response rate surveys do not allow for legitimate comparison from year to year, whereas high response rate surveys generate results that are easy to interpret and difficult to ignore.

• How will you promote the reasons behind the survey? If caregivers are simply handed the survey with no explanation, they will be hesitant to respond openly to questions and may not respond at all. It is key for caregivers to see that leaders are asking these questions because they need the input of frontline staff to be effective stewards of limited quality and safety resources.

• How will you manage the process? Selecting, administering, and responding to a cultural survey is a big job. You may want to establish a steering committee to drive the process. This group would manage selecting the survey instrument, administering the instrument, following up on the results, communicating about the results, capturing the identified issues, and using them to drive improvement.

• How are you going to communicate about results? When you finish the cultural assessment, your work to improve quality has just begun. Usually the senior leadership team is provided the first debriefing of results, followed by the nurse managers/unit directors, and then the frontline staff directly. The most important feedback session is the one you do with frontline staff members, as they are the eyes and ears of safety, and this process provides them a much needed opportunity to engage on a topic that is important to them, in a meaningful way. A best practice for closing the loop on culture assessment while generating next steps that operationalize the results is to conduct a culture debriefing session as outlined in a recent issue of *The Joint Commission Journal on Quality and Patient Safety*™.[21] In this very deliberate process, frontline staff members are given an hour of protected time to complete three basic steps:

1. Review the results and select an item that is particularly relevant to them due to their experience in the clinical area.

2. Envision what the ideal clinical area would look like if 100% of the respondents agreed strongly with the selected item (what processes, norms, behaviors would you see, and what policies would need to be written, or enforced).

3. Identify one actionable step that staff in this clinical area can take to move in the direction of the previously envisioned ideal clinical area (the task, person responsible, follow-up date, and external person or committee to whom the person responsible will hold himself or herself accountable to carry out that step?) This process often identifies dormant safety champions and provides a grass-roots opportunity for caregivers to participate directly in the quality improvement issues important to them.

RESPONDING TO ASSESSMENT DATA

Responding to your cultural assessment data is critical. If you don't respond, you just wasted everyone's time, and you will be unlikely to garner further participation in safety efforts. There are several ways to respond to cultural data:

• Safety culture triage. As previously mentioned, a teamwork or safety climate score with less than 60% agreement signals a clinical area in need of intervention. For example, when fewer than three out of five people agree that safety climate is good in the unit, the lack of consensus indicates substandard clinical and operational outcomes in the eyes of staff, and suggests the need for CUSP[14] or Executive WalkRounds.[17] Conversely, if more than 80% of the caregivers report a good climate, this shows a level of excellence that should be acknowledged by leadership and left to continue unencumbered. (*See* Figures 2-5 and 2-6 on page 18.)

• Taking this concept one step further, you can map low scoring units with inherently dangerous areas, such as the ICU, OR, emergency department, and medical/surgical units with high rates of failure to rescue. By further examining your organization's sentinel event data you can see where poor scores and high risk intersect, and target interventions there, such as daily goals forms, briefings, team training, and so forth. (*See* Figure 2-7 on page 18.) A complete discussion of possible interventions can also be found in Chapters 4–6.

To help with implementation, you can reach out to clinical areas with 80% teamwork climate scores or higher—as they have a consensus of excellence—and ask them to mentor some of the low-performing areas. This breaks down silos within hospitals, and leverages existing strengths to address weaknesses, while respecting the insights and wisdom of frontline staff.

• Determine the cultural success of interventions. By conducting a survey before an intervention and then measuring it again 12–18 months later, you can look for cultural improvement. When measuring the change in safety culture pre- and postintervention, organizations should strive for a 10-point improvement. A 10-point difference between a current assessment and a previous assessment shows a statistically significant difference and demonstrates that your initiative is working.

Figure 2-5. Variability in Teamwork Climate

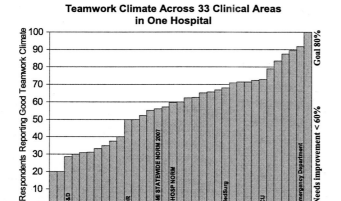

This figure shows one hospital's teamwork climate across 33 clinical areas. Each bar represents the percentage of respondents reporting positive teamwork in their work unit.

Source: Bryan Sexton. Used with permission.

Figure 2-6. Teamwork Collaboration Ratings

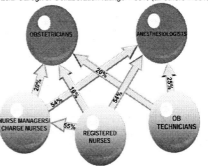

This figure shows the results from the Labor and Delivery Unit in this hospital demonstrated at the level of caregiver role within the clinical area. The ability to "drill down" to find which units are struggling, and which caregiver roles in particular, is a strength of rigorous cultural assessment methodologies.

Source: Bryan Sexton. Used with permission.

Figure 2-7. Recommendations for Improving Teamwork and Safety Climate

TEAMWORK CLIMATE	SAFETY CLIMATE

• Morning/Shift Briefings
• Daily Goals
• Shadowing Exercise
• OR Briefings
• SBAR
• Use Critical Language ("I need some clarity.")
• Simulation
• Team Training
• Culture Checkup Tool
• Reach out within this hospital
  ○ Consult with other clinical areas that have 80% teamwork climate or higher, as they have a consensus of excellence.
	• Executive Partnership Training and Certification Program
	  ○ Use this for your lowest scoring clinical areas first, as it is a powerful intervention, more targeted than traditional Executive WalkRounds™.
	• Hero Form (Feedback from Frontline Workers)
	• Root Cause Life
	• Science of Safety Training
	  ○ 45-minute online course; free registration is required
	  ○ http://distance.jhsph.edu/trams/index.cfm?event=training.launch&trainingID=72
	  ○ Culture Checkup Tool
	• Reach out within this hospital
	  ○ Consult with other clinical areas that have 80% teamwork climate or higher, as they have a consensus of excellence.

This figure shows some possible interventions to help improve teamwork and safety climate. Further discussion of these interventions can be found in Chapters 4–6.

Source: Bryan Sexton. Used with permission.

THE FUTURE OF CULTURAL ASSESSMENT

Most safety culture assessments are being done at the clinical area level. However, researchers are now starting to map relationships between types of caregivers within a clinical area. For example, in obstetrics, how do the nurses relate to each other, the obstetrician, the anesthesiologist, and so forth? By looking at collaboration by caregiver type, we can better match the interventions and next steps to the specific needs of the clinical area. Moreover, case-based climate,[16] where the teamwork during a specific procedure is assessed by all the caregivers present during that procedure, provides even more diagnosticity and is already being used in ORs to understand the impact of preoperative briefings on delays, surgical site and side awareness, and nurse turnover rates.

Safety culture research is still evolving, and those health care systems with multiple years of trend data are pioneers at the bleeding edge of patient safety. Over time, the role of safety culture assessment will increase in importance, as the current health care system is too complex and too unreliable for health care leaders to tackle on their own. They need to be armed with the wisdom of frontline caregivers in their quivers to make significant and sustainable progress.

During the writing of this chapter, Dr. Bryan Sexton was supported by RWJ Foundation grant 58292. Sarah Grillo, Christen Fullwood, and Peter Pronovost have each contributed their considerable perspectives regarding the successful management of survey administrations, and the operational decisions necessary to collect and fully utilize safety culture data. The lessons learned in this journey are due to the profound wisdom of quality, safety, and risk leadership across the 2,000 hospitals where the SAQ has been administered.

REFERENCES

1. Clarke S.: Safety culture on the UK railway network. *Work & Stress* 12:285–292, 1998.
2. Carroll J.: Safety culture as an ongoing process: Culture surveys as opportunities for inquiry and change. *Work & Stress* 12:272–284, 1998.
3. Sexton J., Thomas E.: Measurement: Assessing a safety culture. In Leonard M., Frankel A., Simmonds T. (eds.): *Achieving Safe and Reliable Healthcare strategies and solutions.* Chicago: Health Administration Press, 2004, pp. 115–127.
4. Zohar D.: A group-level model of safety climate: Testing the effect of group climate on microaccidents in manufacturing jobs. *J Appl Psychol* 85:587–596, 2000.
5. Cheyne A., et al.: Modeling safety climate in the prediction of levels of safety activity. *Work & Stress* 12:255–271, 1998.
6. Zohar D.: Safety climate in industrial organizations: Theoretical and applied implications. *J Appl Psychol* 65:96–102, 1980.
7. Donald I., Canter D.: Employee attitudes and safety in the chemical industry. *J Loss Prevention in the Process Industries* 7:203–208, 1994.
8. Dedobbeleer N., Beland F.: A safety climate measure for construction sites. *J Safety Res* 22:97–103, 1991.
9. Niskanen T.: Safety climate in the road administration. *Safe Sci* 17:237–255, 1994.
10. Barling J., Loughlin C., Kelloway E.: Development and test of a model linking transformational leadership and occupational safety. *J Appl Psychol* 87:488–496, 2002.
11. Hofmann D., Stetzer A.: A cross-level investigation of factors influencing unsafe behaviors and accidents. *Personnel Psychology* 49:307–339, 1996.
12. Cooper M., Phillips R.: Exploratory analysis of the safety climate and safety behavior relationship. *J Safety Res* 35:497–512, 2004.
13. Hofmann D., Morgeson F., Gerras S.: Climate as a moderator of the relationship between leader-member exchange and content specific citizenship: Safety climate as an exemplar. *J Appl Psychology* 88:170–178, 2003.
14. Pronovost P.J., et al.: Implementing and validating a comprehensive unit-based safety program. *J Patient Safety* 1:33–40, 2005.
15. DeFontes J., Surbida S.: Preoperative Safety Briefing Project. *The Permanente Journal* 8:21–27, 2004.
16. Makary M.A., et al.: Operating room briefings and wrong-site surgery. *JACS* 204:236–243, Feb 2007.
17. Thomas E.J., et al.: The effect of executive walk rounds on nurse safety climate attitudes: A randomized trial of clinical units. *BMC Health Serv Res* 5:4, Jun. 8, 2005.
18. Pronovost P.J., et al.: Improving patient safety in intensive care units in Michigan. *J Crit Care* 23:207–221, Jun. 2008.
19. Pronovost P.J., Sexton J.B.: Assessing safety culture: Guidelines and recommendations. *Qual Saf Health Care* 14:231–233, 2005.
20. Sexton J.B., et al.: The Safety Attitudes Questionnaire: Psychometric properties, benchmarking data, and emerging research. *BMC Health Services Research* 6:44, Apr. 3, 2006.
21. Sexton J.B., et al.: A culture check-up for safety in "My Patient Care Area." *Jt Comm J Qual Patient Saf* 33:699–703, Nov. 2007.
22. Agency for Healthcare Quality and Research: *Patient Safety Culture Surveys.* http://www.ahrq.gov/qual/hospculture (accessed Jul. 20, 2008).
23. Modak I., et al.: Measuring safety related attitudes in the ambulatory setting: The Ambulatory Safety Attitudes Questionnaire. *JGIM* 22:1–5, Jan. 2007.

Chapter Three

ACCOUNTABILITY AND THE REALITY OF THE HUMAN CONDITION

Allan Frankel, Frank Federico, and *Michael Leonard*

When bad things happen a knee-jerk reaction is to look for someone to blame. When something goes wrong, the common tendency is to find out "who did it" rather than "why." Although this approach is understandable in health care because it makes organizations feel as if they have responded to a problem and taken action, the underlying flaw with this approach is that only about 5% of medical harm is caused by incompetent or poorly intended care, and consequently 95% of errors that cause harm involve conscientious, competent individuals who, through a series of system failures, make a mistake that leads to an unintended and sometimes catastrophic result. Consequently, placing blame on an individual does not address the underlying issues that cause harm and does not prevent the harm from happening again.

Consider this example. A dedicated nurse had 15 years of clinical experience as an obstetrical nurse and spent her entire career working on the obstetrical unit of a large Midwestern hospital. She was integral in creating the hospital's infant bereavement program and was a valued asset to the organization.

The obstetrics unit on which the nurse worked did not use float or traveling nurses, so nurses on the unit filled in extra shifts. To encourage nurses to take extra shifts, the hospital gave an award—a trip to a nursing conference—to the nurse who worked the most overtime hours in a given year. One day in July, the nurse worked a double shift of 16 hours. Because the unit was shorthanded, she agreed to work another shift—laid down for 5–6 hours—and resumed patient care.

Of note was that the hospital had recently installed a new bar-coding system, which was working only about two out of three times, and, according to the nurses, had problems reading IV bags, including those that contained antibiotics and local

anesthetics.

Also, because the obstetrics (OB) unit did not have anesthesia providers dedicated to OB that were based on the unit, the floor nurses had to request an anesthesiologist to come from the operating room area to the OB unit every time a patient needed an epidural—some 2,000 times a year. To help address the inconvenience of this setup, the hospital had a task force of anesthesia and OB unit providers working on a protocol whereby the nurses would prepare the patients, get all the supplies and medications for the epidural analgesia, and have the patient completely ready before the anesthesiologist arrived to place the epidural. This formalized workaround—including laminated reminder cards on the wall—required nurses to pull a medication without a physician's order to save time for the physician. When the physician came to the obstetrics unit, he or she then signed the orders for the drugs the nurse had pulled.

During her shift, the nurse was taking care of two patients: one whose child had died in utero but the patient had not yet given birth, and a 16-year-old having her first baby. Both of these patients required a lot of attention and compassion. The nurse was not only fatigued because of lack of sleep and long, back-to-back shifts, but she was dealing with emotionally charged patients, which was stressful. The teen needed an antibiotic to help treat a strep infection during labor. When the nurse went to hang the IV antibiotic, she accidentally hung a bag of local anesthetic—bupivicaine— which was housed in packaging that was very similar in appearance to the antibiotic. One drug had an orange dot on the bag. The other had a yellow dot. Both drugs were sitting on a table in the patient's room. The bupivicaine had been pulled by another nurse who was preparing to contact the anesthesiologist to give her patient an epidural.

Bupivicaine, a very commonly used local anesthetic, is very cardiotoxic, meaning that a significant IV dose can and will cause cardiac arrest. When the patient seized and suffered acute cardiovascular collapse, the care team emergently focused on getting down the hall to the operating room and delivering the baby by C-section. A normal baby was delivered. Unfortunately, the mother died.

As tragic as the death of a 16-year-old mother is, it was compounded by the fact that the nurse was now facing criminal charges in the patient's death. Despite the myriad system issues that lead to the nurse's mistake—systematically encouraged fatigue, look-alike packaging, ineffective technology that led to workarounds, and an approved process in which nurses pulled medication without a physician's order—the hospital did not view the death as a result of system failures, but placed blame squarely on the shoulders of one of its finest nurses.

In looking at this case objectively, how does blaming the nurse address the problem and prevent it from happening again? The fact is, it does not. Not only does this approach irrevocably alter the nurse's life and career, but it does not address the fundamental system issues that contributed to the mistake. It also eliminates the opportunity to learn from errors—both this one and any future errors—because staff members at the hospital know exactly how errors will be treated and what will happen to them if they admit a mistake.

In addition to the general ineffectiveness of blaming the conscientious employee who makes a mistake, another critically important side effect to this approach is that it creates and reinforces a culture of fear. In this environment, people learn quite quickly to be quiet about problems, mistakes, near misses, and the like because they expect punishment if they speak up. This in turn limits an organization's ability to learn from and address system errors. An adverse event provides insight into the care delivery process, and the open, honest discussion of adverse events is a primary way to truly understand the strengths and weaknesses of care delivery and opportunities for improving flawed policies and practices that increase the risk of error and patient harm.

DEFINING A JUST CULTURE

As mentioned in Chapter 1, one of the most important jobs of organization leadership is to foster a just culture in which everyone knows how the organization will view and respond to errors. It can be said that no other element plays as criti-

cal a role in defining a culture. A just culture is a culture of trust in which people are encouraged to provide essential safety-related information, but in which they are also clear about where the line must be drawn between acceptable and unacceptable behavior.[1] Contrary to popular belief, establishing a just culture is not about removing blame. Removing blame from the workplace does not eliminate individual or organizational responsibility. A just culture is characterized by clear systems thinking, organizational learning, well-developed decision-making mechanisms, and clear organizational structures.[2]

According to one prominent health care organization, "A fair and just culture means giving constructive feedback and critical analysis in skillful ways, doing assessments that are based on facts, and having respect for the complexity of the situation. It also means providing fair-minded treatment, having productive conversations, and creating effective structures that help people reveal their errors and help the organization learn from them."[2]

A health care organization has established a "just culture" when the majority of its members share the belief that justice will be dispensed when the line between acceptable and unacceptable behavior has been crossed. A just culture recognizes that it is unacceptable to punish all errors and unsafe acts, and it is equally unacceptable to provide blanket immunity from sanctions to all actions that could, or did, contribute to harm.

Organizations that are successful in developing and sustaining a just culture are those that have a clear policy statement and framework to guide their response to unsafe acts and adverse outcomes, along with leadership's resolve to create a climate of "psychological safety"[3] and support caregivers who voice concerns.

ESTABLISHING AN ACCOUNTABILITY SYSTEM

To create and foster a just culture, leadership must define, communicate about, and consistently reinforce a system of accountability, which differentiates when good people inadvertently make a mistake because of a series of system issues and when individuals deliberately cause harm or knowingly put a patient at risk without sufficient potential benefit.

Individual accountability must be characterized by clear role definition and relationship delineation.[2] An accountability model enables an organization to promote a just culture that strikes a balance between the benefits of learning at the organizational, interpersonal, and individual levels and the need to retain personal accountability and discipline.[4]

Organizations should pledge within their policies to look objectively at errors and place blame appropriately. Staff members should know that they will be held accountable for their own performance but will not be expected to carry the burden for system flaws. They should know what to expect from the organization when an error occurs and how they will be held accountable. Staff should be assured that the constant goal is systems improvement and decreasing harm to the next patient, and that the act of speaking up will, first and foremost, be used to improve the system of care delivery.

WHY IS AN ACCOUNTABILITY SYSTEM IMPORTANT?

The main reason such an accountability system is critical is that people make mistakes. No matter how skilled, conscientious, well-intentioned, and experienced individuals may be, there are inherent human limitations or factors that make errors possible. Couple that with the fact that care, treatment, and services are often provided amid constant distractions when providers are in a hurry, fatigued, and under pressure, and individuals can overestimate their abilities and underestimate their limitations. They can fail to recognize the impact of factors such as fatigue, stress, and environmental distractions, including noise or poor lighting.

As mentioned in Chapter 1, the culture of many health care organizations is anchored by the belief that if skilled, smart people just try hard and work diligently, they can avoid mistakes and prevent human error. This model of the expert individual is strongly reinforced in the clinical education process. However, this viewpoint is inherently flawed, as humans by their very nature are wired to make mistakes, and no amount of hard work and effort can prevent that.

Errors of commission, such as administering the wrong medication to a patient because it looks or sounds alike another; errors of omission, such as unknowingly skipping a step while programming a medication pump; and even simple arithmetic errors, such as that which may occur when calculating a medication dose, are all part of the human condition and occur with alarming regularity. The fact is people will forget to do something (error of omission) approxi-

mately 1 out of every 100 times they are required to do it. They will do something wrong (an error of commission) approximately 1 out of every 300 times.[5] Consider how many times a nurse must check a drug label in a typical day. Or how many times a physician must write an order for a particular drug. Or how many times a respiratory therapist must administer a particular medication. Now consider that one out of every 100–300 times that nurse will forget to read the label or read it incorrectly; that physician will leave something off of the prescription or write that prescription incorrectly, and that respiratory therapist may forget to administer a medication or administer it incorrectly. How will your organization react to these errors? How you answer that question will help define whether you have a just culture or not.

Factors That Negatively Effect Human Performance

There are many human factors that lead to error in the health care environment. For example, illness, boredom, frustration, and the use of drugs and alcohol can all impair performance and lead to human error. The following sections take a brief look at some of the other human factors that can lead to error:

- Limited Short-Term Memory. The human brain can hold only five to seven pieces of information in short-term memory at one time. Practitioners in a complex environment like medicine deal with a continuous yet frequently interrupted flow of information and tasks over the course of a day—often on a minute-to-minute basis. In fact, observational studies[6] of medical/surgical nurses show they are trying to hold 17–20 items in memory 70% of the time they are at work. Being in a busy environment with information constantly coming in means that an individual's ability to hold, keep track of, prioritize, and manage all the information being received is quickly exceeded. Systems that rely on human memory are highly prone to failure.

- Being late or in a hurry. It is human nature to cut corners when behind or in a hurry. The great majority of the time, cutting corners pays off. The job gets done more quickly or a little bit easier, and there is no apparent downside because errors are rare and the impact of many errors is modest. In fact, individuals are typically rewarded for cutting corners. However, when in a hurry, a person is less selective in his or her attention to details, and the chances of missing something that can contribute to error and possibly cause harm increase significantly. There is a very real danger with cutting corners that over time progressively more corners will be cut without any apparent compromise of safety. The cumulative effect of all these cut corners is called the "normalization of deviance"—when things that are obviously risky become accepted as "we've always done it that way and never had a problem."[7] (*See* Sidebar 3-1, right, for a further discussion of normalization of deviance.)

• Limited Ability to Multitask. Most people, even highly trained ones, are not good multitaskers. Typically individuals are far better at singular task performance. An example of this is people's inability to drive cars safely and talk on cell phones. It is estimated that nearly 3,000 people are injured each year because of cell phone use in their cars.[10] In health care, providers—particularly nurses—are asked to multitask every day. They must check for allergies and administer medication to one patient, while changing a dressing on another patient, while taking vital signs on another patient, and also remember to regularly wash their hands, document information, and communicate effectively. According to a study by Spear and Tucker, nurses perform an average of 100 tasks in an eight-hour shift with a task taking an average of three minutes. They spend time running from task to task to task, and often don't know what the overall plan of care is and thus have a limited ability to prioritize. They are also formally interrupted at least once every hour. As a result of this environment, when a patient has a problem, the nurse is so busy multitasking, he or she may not notice the issue until it has reached a critical level.[11]

• Interruptions. The daily experience in complex environments like medicine is that interruptions are more the norm than the exception. When distracted from tasks considered critically important, even experts require formal cues to get back on track. Interruptions are a huge source of risk, and yet they tend to be regarded as annoyances rather than as the threat they pose. When interrupted, an individual's ability to get back on task is dependent on short-term memory, which, as previously discussed, is quite limited.

• Stress. Human factors research consistently demonstrates that error rates increase with significant stress. Individuals have a 30% chance of making an error when highly stressed as opposed to a 0.1% chance when not stressed. When under stress, there is increased likelihood that individuals will shift from rapid, accurate expert deci-

---

Sidebar 3-1. The Difference Normalization of Deviance[8]

The *normalization of deviance* is a term authored by Diane Vaughn in her analysis of the 1986 *Challenger* space shuttle accident. It refers to the accumulated effect of cutting corners over time. While the effect of each of these shortcuts individually is usually not significant, when added together, what is considered safe and reasonable can be changed dramatically. Very typically, the normalization of deviance leaves everyone shaking their heads in the aftermath of an accident and asking, "How did we get here?"

In the case of the *Challenger* disaster, over a period of 24 launches in the NASA Shuttle program, the minimum safe launch temperature incrementally moved from 55 degrees Fahrenheit to 36 degrees on the January day in 1986 when the O-rings failed. Slowly, over time, these numerous small reductions in the safe launch temperature pushed the envelope of safety.

The loss of the *Columbia* space shuttle in 2003 resulted from a similar problem. During many previous shuttle flights, foam insulation fell from the external fuel tank during liftoff. These flights were seemingly unaffected by the debris and thus the problem was ignored. Unfortunately, on February 1, 2003, the falling insulation damaged the shuttle's left wing and was the physical cause of the tragedy. According to the *Chicago Tribune*, the pressure to keep on schedule led NASA to habitually accept the persistent problem of the falling foam and come to view it as normal.[7,9]

Though the technical term Diane Vaughn applied to the *Challenger* launch decision was "The Normalization of Deviance", a common, practical term to describe the accumulated result of many shortcuts is "drift."

---

sion making to an inefficient, slow, conscious problem-solving process that is highly error-prone. For example, under normal circumstances, a provider can successfully select and pick out the correct medication vial 99.9% of the time. However, when performing the same task in a very stressful situation, such as the middle of a cardiac arrest, the error rate can be as high as 25%, a 250-fold increase![5]

Stress is also a likely contributor toward tunnel vision—not being able to see the forest for the trees. People who are stressed can easily become "tunnel-visioned" and lose sight of the bigger picture. They also tend to revert to previous patterns of behavior and are more likely to filter information in ways that fit the desired end result. This tendency greatly increases the chances that conclusions are wrong. If an individual makes the wrong choice initially, the danger is he or she will selectively filter incoming information to verify his or her initial decision, and discard critical data that reveal something else is going on.

Consider this unfortunate and true example. An anesthesiologist is putting a healthy patient to sleep. Everything is going smoothly, and the anesthesiologist is easily ventilating the patient using a mask. However, when the endotracheal breathing tube is placed, the patient has extreme difficulty breathing. The pressure required to deliver a breath is alarmingly high; the end-tidal CO_2 monitor—the gold standard used to verify the integrity of a patient's breathing—reads zero; and the patient's oxygen saturation falls to life-threatening levels. Not considering the possibility that the breathing tube is in the wrong place— the leading cause of anesthetic death in healthy patients—the physician interprets the situation as an indicator of an acute, massive asthma attack. The absence of carbon dioxide on the monitor is attributed to abrupt failure of the device, which has worked well for the anesthesiologist on three prior cases that day.

In reality, the patient's breathing tube has been mistakenly placed in the esophagus, and the anesthesiologist, not recognizing the potentially lethal error, persists in reading the incoming data into his very tenuous construct. The critical error in this case is not placing the tube incorrectly—it happens to the best of clinicians— but not recognizing the problem and fixing it. If the anesthesiologist had thought, "Things were great until the tube was placed, and then the problem began. Let's take the tube out and see if things get better," this situation would have been a nonevent. However, the failure to consider a possible mistake and the refusal to interpret overwhelmingly obvious information indicating that the tube is in the wrong place does great harm.[7]

• Lack of Sleep and Fatigue. Each year, millions of Americans progress through life tired. Nearly 40% of the workforce in this country experiences fatigue on the job,[12] and nearly 70% of the American public does not get enough sleep during the week.[13] In the often fast-paced world of health care, worker fatigue has always been a potential patient safety and provider safety risk. Fatigue has been linked to decreases in performance and increases in medical errors and workplace accidents.

Fatigue can have a detrimental effect on cognitive ability, specifically the ability to process complex information. The working assumption that motivation and skill can overcome inherent physiologic limitations of fatigue is a dangerous one. It has been shown that cognitive performance after 24 hrs without sleep is equivalent to performance with a blood alcohol level of 0.10.[14] Research also shows that sleep debt is cumulative and the physiologic effects will persist until enough sleep has been obtained to pay it back.[15]

Fatigue can impact physicians' and nurses' technical skills and their ability to perform specific procedures. For example, studies have shown that surgeons have less surgical dexterity and operate more slowly when fatigued.[16] Whether administering an intravenous (IV) medication or monitoring a patient during anesthesia, degradation of attention, memory, and coordination due to fatigue can affect performance, impact patient safety, and lead to adverse events.[17] Mistakes caused by fatigue are most likely to occur during routine tasks and those that require sustained concentration. Effects on urgent tasks or those that require short yet significant bursts of mental energy are less. Often, fatigue-related mistakes involve the failure to recognize the existence of a serious problem. For example, giving the wrong antibiotic to a septic patient is not typically a fatigue-related mistake; however, failing to recognize that altered mental status might represent sepsis is typical of a fatigue-related error.[18]

Interestingly enough, fatigue causes fewer performance problems in workers with more control over their work because they can schedule nonurgent tasks or tasks that require sustained concentration for periods when they are at their best. Physicians will thus cope better with fatigue than staff members with less job flexibility, such as nurses.[18]

In addition to the patient safety risks associated with fatigue, there are several provider safety risks. Physical and mental health, interpersonal relationships, and the ability to perform the tasks of daily life can all be affected by acute sleep loss and fatigue. In addition to detrimental health effects, there is a well-documented connection between fatigue and an increased likelihood of on-the-job accidents.[19] Some of those accidents may include needlestick injuries and bloodborne pathogen exposure. One recent study found that the number of hours worked per day, the number of weekends worked per month, and whether individuals worked evening and night shifts were significantly associated with needlestick injuries.[20]

Fatigue is not only a contributor to workplace accidents, but accidents that occur outside the workplace as well. According to one study, first-year medical interns who work shifts longer than 24 hours are more than twice as likely as interns who work shorter shifts to be in a car crash after leaving work, and five times as likely to have a near-miss.[21] Studies also report increased rates of crashes in nurses when driving home after working a night shift.[22] Another study showed that 24% of residents surveyed reported falling asleep driving home since becoming a physician, 66% had felt close to falling asleep at the wheel in the past 12 months, and 42% recalled a fatigue-related clinical error in the past 6 months.[23]

• The Detrimental Effects of Shift Work. Hospitals function around the clock and therefore require shift work. Typically, shift work is performed outside the daytime hours of 7 A.M. to 6 P.M. and includes evening shifts, night shifts, rotating shifts, and on-call shifts. More than 20% of the U.S. workforce participates in shift work, and approximately 30% of nurses employed in full-time health care engage in this type of work.[24] In health care, individuals who participate in shift work or who engage in prolonged work hours—such as shifts lasting 12 hours or more—are more likely to be fatigued than those who work a more regular schedule. Evening and night-shift workers can be particularly susceptible to fatigue. Human beings are biologically wired to be awake during the day and asleep at night, and work schedules that oppose this natural rhythm can generate physiologic disruptions that lead to significantly degraded performance and increased risks to health and safety.[25] Physicians-in-training who work traditional schedules with recurrent 24-hour shifts greatly increase the risk of injuring their patients or others and incur the following risks[26]:

• Make 36% more serious medical errors than those whose scheduled work is limited to 15 consecutive hours

• Make five times as many serious diagnostic errors

• Have twice as many on-the-job attention failures at night

• Suffer 61% more needlestick and other sharp injuries after 20 consecutive hours of work

• Report making 300% more fatigue-related medical errors that lead to a patient's death

A recent study, which surveyed residents about medical errors, found that the odds of reporting at least one fatigue-related clinically significant medical error increased by a factor of 7 during months in which the residents worked five or more overnight shifts, as compared with months in which

they worked no overnight shifts.[27] The study showed that interns made 35.9% more serious medical errors when they worked frequent shifts of 24 hours or more—a more traditional schedule—than when they worked shorter shifts. They also made 56.6% more nonintercepted serious errors and 5.6 times as many serious diagnostic errors during the traditional schedule. Consequently, the study showed that eliminating extended work shifts and reducing the number of hours interns work per week can reduce serious medical errors.[27]

Nurses encounter similar shift work–related fatigue risks. A study of nurses showed that the risk of a nurse making an error significantly increased when the nurse's work shift exceeded 12 hours, when overtime was worked, or when work hours exceeded more than 40 hours per week. In fact, the likelihood of a nurse making an error was three times higher when the shift lasted 12.5 hours or more. This study also indicated that many nurses work past their scheduled shift time, and those individuals who did work past their 12-hour-shift were most vulnerable for making an error.[28]

• Environmental Factors. Environmental factors, such as heat, noise, visual stimuli, distractions, and lighting can all adversely affect human performance and lead to mistakes. Environmental distractions can be seen in operating rooms, which are frequently noisy with music playing, patient monitors beeping, and conversations going on. In addition, there are electrical cords on the floor and various tubes and gas lines present. From an ergonomic engineering point of view, the array, or more appropriately, disarray of equipment, is a chaotic nightmare. In addition, many operating room doors are barely wide enough to accommodate a patient bed going in or out. Workplace design is an integral part of keeping patients and staff safe.

System Errors and Latent Failures

In addition to human factors that lead to human error, system malfunctions, limitations, and breakdowns can also lead to error. Also know as "latent errors," these might include poorly designed workflow, incorrect installation of equipment, faulty maintenance, and poor organizational structure. In health care, frontline providers are so used to design defects resulting from latent errors that they learn to work around them. These workarounds can also lead to error because safety steps are often skipped or overlooked. It is essential to have a good understanding of complex systems, and latent and active failures when building a model of accountability. James Reason's work is a great place to start. Go to http://www.bmj.com/cgi/reprint/320/7237/768.pdf for more information on Reason's work.[1]

Both human and latent system errors do not always lead to harm. Many times providers will notice problems in situations and address them before they cause harm. Other errors do reach the patient, but, because of the resiliency of the human body among other factors, don't cause harm. However, the combination of human factors and system issues can sometimes create the "perfect storm" in health care with the patient in the eye of the storm. It is in this perfect storm that we see a majority of preventable adverse outcomes, and it is the navigation of this storm that requires an accountability system.

HOW TO CREATE A JUST ACCOUNTABILITY SYSTEM

Creating an accountability system does not have to be challenging. Although there are many ways to create such a system, one easy way is to base it on James Reason's five-part algorithm, which involves asking the following questions whenever an error occurs:

1. Was there malicious intent? Did the individual intentionally engage in activity to cause harm?

2. Was the person knowingly impaired? For example, was he or she intoxicated or under the influence of an unauthorized substance, such as illicit drugs? Was there a medical illness that impaired his or her judgment?

3. Did the individual do something he or she knew was wrong or knowingly unsafe? For example, was the person knowingly violating safe operating procedure, such as refusing to engage in a presurgical time-out to verify the correct patient, procedure, and site?

4. Did the individual make a mistake someone of similar training would make? For example, if a patient in the emergency department has a grossly abnormal electrocardiogram, and the physician sends him home where he suffers a heart attack and dies, the question becomes would another physician have made the same mistake given the system issues present at the time?

5. Is the individual involved a "frequent flier"—has he or she been involved in multiple adverse events? Has he or she been repeatedly involved in similar events?

Within Reason's model, the first three components reveal violations at an individual level and indicate that the individual should be held accountable for his or her actions. The fourth question is sometimes referred to as the substitution test and can indicate whether there is an individual issue or a system error. If two to three peers would make a similar mistake given the circumstances, then the error can be attributed to system issues. However, if an individual's peers would not make such a mistake then it raises questions of technical skill, training, and judgment.

The fifth question, which deals with repeat participants, raises significant issues as to judgment and knowledge. Can these be mitigated with training and education? People who have been involved multiple times in similar events are less likely to be good candidates for training and education. If an organization concludes that these types of interventions do not have a likelihood of success, they do have a nonnegotiable obligation to provide safe care. In these instances, these individuals may need to be changed to a different role.

Let's go back to the example at the beginning of this chapter. In asking the five questions about the veteran nurse who made a mistake, which led to the death of a teenage girl, how would you classify the error?

• Was there malicious intent? Did the nurse intentionally engage in activity to cause harm? No.

• Was the nurse knowingly impaired? For example, was she intoxicated or under the influence of an unauthorized substance, such as illicit drugs? Was there a medical illness that impaired her judgment? No.

• Did the individual do something she knew was wrong or knowingly unsafe? Although the nurse did obtain drugs without a physician's order, this was tacitly sanctioned by the organization as part of a performance improvement initiative. Did she engage in conscious risk taking by not using the bar-coding system? We would need to know whether it was available, working, and how many other nurses were working around it. If this was common behavior on the unit, it is hard to hold one nurse accountable. If she was the only one, that changes the conversation.

• Did the individual make a mistake someone of similar training would make? Yes. If one of her peers was fatigued, stressed, in a hurry, working around a poorly functioning technology, and following a protocol that was inherently flawed just as this nurse was, the likelihood the peer would make the same mistake is great.

- Had she been involved in similar events? No.

Although James Reason's model is not the only way to establish an accountability system, it provides a clear-cut and straightforward way to start the process. By incorporating some version of Reason's algorithm into your organization's accountability system, you can deal with most accountability questions very quickly. It is critically important that the caregiver at the bedside be able to ask himself or herself a very short list of questions in the aftermath of an error or near miss to determine his or her level of accountability and know it is safe to tell someone about the event, so the situation can likely be remedied to prevent it from happening again. It is also important that the organization has only "one set of rules," applied consistently and openly to everyone regardless of their standing in the organization or the severity of the event.

In addition to Reason's model, David Marx, an engineer and lawyer, has elegantly applied an engineering perspective to accountability and developed a Just Culture Algorithm that has become quite popular in the United States. The algorithm has as its foundation the concept that individuals should be held accountable for the choices they make. Marx has taken this tack because the provision of health care, especially among physicians, has tended toward a perspective of "no harm, no foul"—in other words even if an action is reckless, if no damage occurs, organizations are willing to turn a blind eye to the activity.

Marx divides actions into three categories to support this framework. Actions deemed blameless occur when individuals inadvertently make mistakes or errors. The causes of these have been aptly described in this chapter and are a result of human fallibility, especially in complex environments.

The algorithm then delves into an aspect of decision making that Reason's indecision tree hints at in his substitution test—when he asks whether other similarly skilled and trained individuals would perform in the same way as the individual being evaluated—but the substitution test only hints at a concept that Marx delves into in great detail. Marx describes the other two categories of actions as "at-risk" behavior and "reckless" behavior and is quick to point out that differentiation between the two can be made only through the lens of what the culture—the local society—perceives as allowable. An example helps to clarify this

nuanced issue. Take hand washing. Today, most would agree that choosing to not wash hands prior to touching a patient is blatant reckless behavior. Indeed, if the hospital deems hand hygiene noncompliance as reckless and responds accordingly by uniform sanctions when noncompliance occurs, individuals will be on notice to carefully wash their hands, and other than the occasional mistake where a clinician forgets or is distracted while entering a patient's room, (all blameless and allowable omission errors) exceptions to good hand washing will be forbidden and noncompliance will be, to all, reckless behavior. However, if a hospital deems hand hygiene noncompliance as reckless yet doesn't respond when individuals knowingly ignore the rules, then, by cultural norm, omitting washing hands is "at-risk" behavior. Organizations that then arbitrarily sanction clinicians only by outcome, when patients become infected, are acting erratically—and destined to be perceived by their employees and clinicians as untrustworthy. The effect is to stymie efforts that promote transparency and learning because individuals are unsure of the response they'll receive. The clinician is accountable for at-risk behavior, and the organization is accountable for poorly upholding its standards of care.

Marx describes a just culture as one that "recognizes that while we as humans are fallible, we do generally have control of our behavioral choices, whether we are an executive, a manager, or a staff member. Just Culture flourishes in an organization that understands the concept of shared accountability—that good system design and good behavioral choices of staff together produce good results. It has to be both."[29]

RELENTLESSLY REINFORCE THE MESSAGE

Before implementing an accountability system, it may be helpful to determine the staff's familiarity with the concept of a nonpunitive culture. Both frontline staff and managers must be clear on what is expected from them and how they will be held accountable for errors.

After leaders have established an accountability system, they can't just mention it once and forget it, they must continuously educate, reinforce, and demonstrate their commitment to consistent accountability and learning from mistakes. This can't be stressed enough. Because accountability is a critical element in the creation and maintenance of a safe culture, organization leadership must commit to an accountability system and consistent application of that system across the organization. Some ways to do this include the following:

• Create policies and procedures that support the accountability system and the entire error management process. Such policies should be shared with staff and leadership.

• Educate frontline staff on the accountability system. This education needs to be wall-to-wall. All staff should be educated on the policy and see consistent reinforcement of it by leadership. Education can take many forms, including during staff meetings, within Executive WalkRounds (*see* Chapter 5), during online training sessions, and so forth. Such education should change these staff perspectives:

—That was a weak moment. I won't do it again.

—I am absolutely not going to tell anyone, because I will get in big trouble.

—Why should I tell them? Nothing will change.

• Educate staff on human factors and their contributions to medical error. This type of education must combat the previously mentioned cultural tendency to assume that through hard work and commitment, errors can be avoided. Staff members should be aware of the human factors that contribute to error and be able to recognize those factors in their work life. They also should feel comfortable reporting situations in which human factors have the potential to cause errors and work to redesign processes to mitigate the effects of those factors. For example, to help combat the effects of fatigue, some organizations are instituting a planned nap program for individuals who work the night shift. In most cases, the nap is voluntary. Staff must learn the effects of fatigue on performance, recognize the signs of fatigue, and feel empowered to take a planned nap when necessary.

• Make the accountability system part of the orientation process for new hires as well as the continuing education program for current staff.

• Educate managers on the accountability system. Middle management must understand the algorithm, know how to use it, and be held accountable for using it consistently. Your organization may want to use scenarios or case examples to help train managers so that they can get practice in consistently using the algorithm. If an event does not neatly fit within the algorithm, managers should be sup-

ported with a senior-level management group that helps navigate grey areas.

• Use real case examples to both educate and reinforce the accountability model—the best ones are your own events. Real cases are very powerful, as many clinicians will have already heard about the event through the rumor mill, and this is a golden opportunity for leaders to model the desired approach to analyzing these events. Not only does it show consistency, but also teaches people about system error and illustrates the organizational commitment to safe care.

• Senior leadership must publicly embrace the accountability system and hold middle management accountable for using it. In a case where a high-profile error goes public, senior leadership must support the participants in the error and avoid the temptation to place blame.

• Create a process in which you learn from errors. As previously mentioned, adverse events provide a unique opportunity for learning. After an event occurs and it is determined to be a system error, your organization should have a consistent process of learning from that error. This should involve looking at contributing factors, such as human factors, environmental considerations, faulty equipment, and so forth. Often, organizations will use a root cause analysis for this process, which is a step-by-step approach to analyzing an error, determining the primary cause(s) of the error, and working to put improvements in place to address the error. More information about root cause analysis can be found in Chapter 13.

As previously mentioned, a key element in an effective accountability system is consistency. The system must be applied the same way every time there is an error. It takes only one case in which a CEO places blame on a frontline provider for a system error, and the entire accountability system and culture of safety is seriously jeopardized as a result of the fragile trust built between staff and leadership being shattered.

A good accountability model is the essential foundation of a functional and safe organizational culture. When caregivers know that there is a transparent set of rules that apply to everyone, and that roughly 95% of the time following an adverse event the individuals involved are recognized as conscientious, highly skilled individuals trying hard to do the right thing, then caregivers will know they are safe to report and discuss errors. This transparency and accountability also allow your organization to say to staff, patients and families;

the media; and regulators that the people who provide care in your organization are capable, conscientious, and trying very hard to do the right things for every patient every day. It is absolutely essential for caregivers to feel safe; otherwise, they never really believe the organization can keep patients safe.

REFERENCES

1. Reason J.T.: *Managing the Risks of Organizational Accidents.* Brookfield, VT: Ashgate; 1997.

2. Connor M., et al.: Creating a fair and just culture: One organization's path toward organizational change. *Jt Comm J Qual Patient Saf* 33:617–624, Oct. 2007.

3. Edmondson A.C.: The competitive imperative of learning. *Harv Bus Rev* 86:7–8, 60–67, Jul.–Aug. 2008.

4. Marx D.: *Patient Safety and the "Just Culture": A Primer for Health Care Executives.* New York City: Columbia University, 2001.

5. Salvendy G.: *Handbook of Human Factors and Ergonomics,* 3rd ed. Hoboken, NJ: Wiley, 2005.

6. Potter P., et al.: Understanding the cognitive work of nursing in the acute care environment. *J Nurs Adm* 35:327–335, Jul.–Aug. 2005.

7. Leonard M., Frankel A. Focusing on high reliability. In Leonard M., Frankel A., Simmonds T. (eds.): *Achieving Safe and Reliable Healthcare: Strategies and Solutions.* Chicago: Health Administration Press, 2004, pp. 15–34.

8. Vaughan D.: *The Challenger Launch Decision: Risky Technology, Culture, and Deviance at NASA.* Chicago: University of Chicago Press, 1996.

9. Kunerth, J., Cabbage, M.: NASA's safety culture blamed. *Chicago Tribune,* Aug. 27, 2003, pp. 1, 26.

10. Cohen J.T., Graham J.D.: A revised economic analysis of restrictions on the use of cell phones while driving. *Risk Anal* 23:5–17, 2003.

11. Tucker A.L., Spear S.J.: Operational failures and interruptions in hospital nursing. *Health Serv Res* 41:643–662, Jun. 2006.

12. Fatigue in the workplace is common and costly. *Medical News Today* http://www.medicalnewstoday.com/medicalnews.php?newsid=60732 (accessed Jul. 15, 2008).

13. National Sleep Foundation: *Sleep in America Poll.* http://www.sleepfoundation.org/atf/cf/%7Bf6bf2668-a1b4-4fe8-8d1a a5d39340d9cb%7D/2008%20POLL%20SOF.PDF (accessed Jul. 15, 2008).

14. Baker A., Simpson S., Dawson D.: Sleep disruption and mood changes associated with menopause. *J Psychosom Res* 43:359–369, 1997.

15. Dinges D.F.: Sleep debt and scientific evidence. *Sleep* 27:1050–1052, Sep. 15, 2004.

16. Eastridge B.J., et al.: Effects of sleep deprivation on the performance of simulated laparoscopic surgical skill. *Am J Surg* 186:169–174, Aug. 2003.

17. Jha A.K., Duncan B.W., Bates D.W.: Fatigue, sleepiness, and medical errors. In Shojania K.G., et al. (eds.): *Making Health Care Safer: A Critical Analysis of Patient Safety Practices.* Evidence Report/Technology Assessment No. 43. Rockville, MD: Agency for Healthcare Research and Quality, 2001, pp. 519–533.

18. Olson L., Ambrogetti A.: Working harder—Working dangerously? Fatigue and performance in hospitals *Med J Aust* 168:614–616, 1998.

19. Fatigue in healthcare workers. HRC Supplement A: Risk Analysis Employment Issues 14. *ECRI* Jan. 2006.

20. Trinkoff A.M., et al.: Work schedule, needle use, and needlestick injuries among registered nurses. *Infect Control Hosp Epidemiol* 28:156–164, Feb. 2007.

21. Barger L.K., et al.: Extended work shifts and the risk of motor vehicle crashes among interns. *N Engl J Med* 13:125–134, Jan. 13, 2005.

22. Caruso C., Condon M.: Night shifts and fatigue: Coping skills for the working nurse. *Am J Nurs* 106:88, Aug. 2006.

23. Gander P., et al.: Work patterns and fatigue-related risk among junior doctors, *Occup Environ Med.* 64:733–738, Mar. 2007

24. Blachowicz E., Letizia M.: The challenges of shift work. *Medsurg Nursing* 15:274–280, Oct. 2006.

25. Managing work schedules: An alertness and safety perspective. In Kryger M.A., Roth T., Dement W.C. (eds.): *Principles and Practice of Sleep Medicine.* Philadelphia: Elsevier Saunders, 2005.

26. Lockley S., et al.: Effects of health care provider work hours and sleep deprivation on safety and performance. *Jt Comm J Qual Patient Saf* 33:7–18, Nov. 2007.

27. Barger L.K., et al.: Impact of extended-duration shifts on medical errors, adverse events, and attentional failures. *PLoS Med* 3:e487, 2006.

28. Rogers A.E., et al.: The working hours of hospital staff nurses and patient safety *Health Aff* 23:202–212, Jul.–Aug. 2004.

29. Marx D., Comden S.C., Sexhus Z.: Our inaugural issue—In recognition of a growing community. *The Just Culture Community News and Views* Nov.–Dec. 2005.

Chapter Four

RELIABILITY AND RESILIENCE

Roger Resar, Frank Federico, Doug Bonacum, **and** *Carol Haraden*

Health care in the United States is one of the most complex systems in existence. Within the health care system, multiple specialized disciplines interact with each other as well as with sophisticated equipment to perform complex procedures in a fast-paced environment. Both the number and type of interacting factors at play can be mind boggling, and the way health care is provided can change from day to day and patient to patient. The complexity and lack of predictability inherent in health care places a premium on reliability—both in processes and in the overall goals of an organization.

WHAT IS RELIABILITY?

In simplest terms, reliability is the probability that a system will consistently perform as designed. It's putting your key in the ignition of your car and being certain it will start; it's knowing that the newspaper is going to be delivered to your door without you having to do anything; it's turning on the TV at night and knowing the news will start exactly at the top of the hour.

Berwick and Nolan defined reliability for health care as "the capability of a process, procedure, or health service to perform its intended function in the required time under commonly existing conditions.[1]" In terms of the aspirations of most health care organizations today, reliability is about providing the right care, to the right patient, at the right time . . . every time. While this may seem obvious, McGlynn et al. have reported that patients actually receive only about 55% of the "right" care and preventive therapy that they should. McGlynn et al. calculated that number by multiplying the reliabilities of each process step together—for example, a 16-step process with a 95.7% per step reliability will achieve an overall 55% success rate (0.957).[2] The importance of this concept in these calculations is that the complexity of delivering care requires many steps to achieve a goal—and each step's intrinsic error rate affects the overall success of the effort. Human limitation and failures ensure that every step has an intrinsic error and failure rate.

Mathematically, reliability might be thought of as the number of actions that achieve an intended result divided by the total number of actions taken:

$$\text{Reliability (system)} = \frac{(\text{\# of actions that achieve an intended result})}{\text{Total number of actions taken}}$$

The reliability of a process or system can also be thought of as the opposite of its rate of error or failure. For example, when a system has an error rate of 1 in 10, it is operating at a level of reliability of 90%. When the error or defect rate is 1 in 100, the level of reliability is 99%. For many processes in health care, achieving an overall reliability rate of approximately 95% would result in remarkably more patient-centered, effective, and efficient care. For other processes, such as administering medication, even a 99% rate of reliability, would be disastrous. In the labeling of laboratory specimens, a 99.9% success rate is inadequate to safeguard patients.

WHY DO ORGANIZATIONS STRUGGLE WITH RELIABILITY?

With all the good intentions and talent available in medicine, why are clinical processes backed by solid medical evidence carried out at such low levels of reliability? Certainly, few people come to work with the intention of performing poorly. The following common themes may offer a partial explanation for the reliability gap:

• Current improvement methods in health care depend excessively on asking people to "pay more attention," "slow down," and "try harder." As discussed in Chapter 3, humans make mistakes, and asking them to pay more attention or try harder won't prevent that from happening. This approach is akin to asking yourself not to forget where you put your car keys or where you parked in a large parking lot . . . ever. While it may be effective every once in awhile, you still are going to misplace your keys or forget where you parked your car, no matter how hard you try.

• The focus on individual outcomes tends to exaggerate reliability. As discussed in Chapter 1, one reason that high error rates have not stimulated more concern and efforts at error prevention may be lack of individual practitioner awareness of the problem. Although error rates are substantial, serious injuries due to errors are not part of the everyday experience of physicians and nurses, and most errors do no harm—they are either intercepted through another individual's vigilance, often the patients, or if they do reach the patient, by serendipity, their effects are nil or minor. For example, few children die from a single misdiagnosed or mistreated urinary infection, and many times nurses don't completely follow the "five rights" of medication administration, yet their patients still get the right dose of the right medication via the right route at the right time. Interestingly enough, because patients don't have easy access to hospital mortality data, hand hygiene compliance, or various hospital-specific surgical complication rates, we have lulled them into having a false sense of security as well. When organizations compare themselves to top-performing organizations, they can more clearly see how their performance needs to improve.

• Clinical autonomy allows wide performance margins. Autonomy, describes Dr. Jim Reinertsen,[3] is that which stands between the great respect for evidence-based medicine and its implementation. In many health care organizations, clinicians have different approaches to care and prefer to be autonomous in how they provide care. One significant consequence of autonomy is unnecessary variation. Unnecessary variation adds complexity to an already complex system, complexity adds ambiguity, and ambiguity creates gaps between what we know and what we do. Unfortunately, our passion for fixing the problem is often trumped by a passion to fight for autonomy, so improvement is severely limited.

• Organizations fail to respond to errors in a manner that prevents recurrence. As discussed in Chapter 3, physicians and nurses are socialized throughout their training to strive for error-free practice. Errors come to be viewed as serious professional failures, often in character—the perception being that the individual "wasn't careful enough." These misguided concepts of infallibility inhibit learning from mistakes, create fear, and result in corrective action that includes a lot of hand-wringing from management regarding what the practitioner "should have" done.

• Processes are rarely designed to meet specific goals. Often organizations redesign processes with no specific goals for performance of the process. When designing a process it's important to set clear targets for reliability. For example, stating that a new process is going to work 95% of the time is an appropriate reliability target because achieving 95% reliability is a reachable goal that doesn't necessarily require significant resources or technology.

DESIGNING FOR RELIABILITY

A first step in achieving reliability in your organization is to design and implement reliable processes and systems. Industries in which many lives rest upon performing every single task that's required, again and again, such as airlines and nuclear power plants, are famous for designing high-reliability processes and systems. Reliable design assists in preventing behaviors and conditions that lead to harm by creating an articulated and workable process that is readily followed and prevents conditions that increase risk due to human factors issues.

To help with reliable design, the Institute for Healthcare Improvement (IHI) has created an approach to redesigning daily workflows that can serve as a foundation to prevent harm from occurring as a result of error. The following sections discuss IHI's approach.

The Prep Work

Prior to redesigning for reliability, there are some "setup" steps required. Failure to set up improvement or redesign projects properly will, at best, delay meaningful change by months, but may, at worst, doom the project. The first step is to select a process that is noncatastrophic to improve. This means that failure to reliably carry out this process does not lead to death or serious injury within a short time period. A noncatastrophic process could be the delivery of preoperative antibiotics. Although potentially harmful if not done reliably, imminent death or serious harm to the patient is not a foregone conclusion. Conversely, operating on the wrong surgical site would be a

Figure 4-1. Three-Step Design Strategy

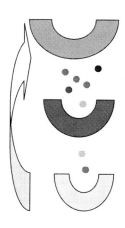

- Step 1: Simplification, standardization, and intent are used to help minimize the chance of process failure.

- Step 2: "Controls" are applied to help prevent error from occurring in the simplified process.

- Step 3: Errors that nevertheless occur are identified and interrupted before they cause harm.

Study the failures and redesign for exceptions if cost/benefit makes sense.

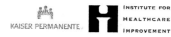

This figure shows the three steps to reliable design. The half circles reflect the levels of redundancy, and the dots illustrate that fewer defects are getting through. The arrow shows the need to have feedback to further improve.

Source: Doug Bonacum, Kaiser Permanente. Used with permission.

catastrophic error because after the error occurs there is no way it can be undone, and irrevocable harm or death is assured. Any clinical practice that is so critical that failure would lead to certain death or serious disability must be redesigned in a more robust way, such as by using Six Sigma methodology. (*See* Chapter 12 for more information on Six Sigma.)

After a process has been selected, the improvement team must choose a segment of the process on which to test redesigns. It is important when segmenting to choose a segment that has a high enough volume so that study of changes reaps adequate information for analysis. The chosen segment should also provide a high probability of success for the types of changes that may be tested. For example, it may be appropriate and helpful to test a process on a particular unit or units, a particular patient population, or on a particular aspect of the process.

After selecting a segment, your organization should map the process, identifying the various failure modes in the process and determining which is the highest priority or greatest leverage point to work on initially. A target for im-

provement should be determined. As previously mentioned, in most cases, 95% reliability is an appropriate target.

The Design Work

The goal of the redesign work is to create processes that are clear, are easy to apply and understand, and can be routinely measured for reliable application by team members. There are three basic steps in designing an everyday practice for reliability.

1. Simplify and standardize to reach 80% reliability.
2. Apply controls to achieve 95% reliability.
3. Identify and interrupt to achieve continuous process improvement.

(*See* Figure 4-1, above, for an illustration of the three-step design strategy and Figure 4-2 on page 37 for a checklist to help navigate the process.)

Step 1: Simplification and Standardization

The goal of step 1 is to achieve a level of reliability in terms of process output that is on the order of 80%–90%. Because many processes in health care involve multiple individuals performing multiple steps in several ways—some of those steps being unnecessary—standardization and simplification can help achieve this first level of reliability.

Simplification is needed to reduce confusion and minimize waste. It is also needed to improve the inherent reliability of the system. At its core, simplification in process flow is about eliminating the unnecessary steps that increase the likelihood of error. The more steps involved in a process, the more likely there will be an error in that process. For example, if a process has one step that is reliably performed 95% of the time, there is a 95% chance that an individual will perform it correctly. Conversely, there is a 5% chance that the individual will perform it incorrectly. While this is pretty low risk for a single-step process, for each additional step in a process, the chances of error compound, so that by the time you have a 40-step process, there is only a 12% chance that all 40 steps in the process will be performed correctly. By simplifying the number and complexity of steps, you reduce the likelihood of error.

After unnecessary steps are eliminated, the next goal is to standardize the simplified process. Why is this important? A single standardized process allows consistency and improves efficiency. Unfortunately, standardization is seldom done well in health care. Most clinical processes have a range of possible ways to accomplish a given task, and all these ways fall within the scope of acceptable medical practice. For years, clinicians have agreed that if there is a single standard based on good medical science, standardization is warranted. However, very few of these clinical opportunities exist. The difficulty with allowing any acceptable process within the scope of practice is related to the lack of infrastructure to support multiple competing processes. For example, multiple approaches to potassium administration in the intensive care unit (ICU) can be problematic. The ability of the ICU to train all nurses and pharmacists in multiple approaches is limited. It involves training new employees in all of the approaches, following up on skills for current staff, coordinating which physicians desire which approaches, and following up on the efficacy of any one approach. By standardizing to one process, organizations can increase efficiency, reduce staff time, and ensure consistency. A single standardized care process allows the institutional expectation of training all the staff in the single protocol and following up on the efficacy of a single protocol.

One of the major benefits in standardizing care is that it helps to create a learning environment. The multiple methods approach makes the recognition of system defects difficult and the correction of defects in a particular protocol even more difficult. Standardization allows the detection of defects from the standardized care process and tracing the defect back to the cause. Each defect then becomes an opportunity to learn and improve the process.

Methods of Standardization

No standardized process can be expected to be successful if isolated experts try to develop the perfect protocol without actually testing it in the clinical environment. Typically, a standardized protocol or care process is written by a group of experts in a nonexperiential setting, making an attempt to compromise and account for all possible objections and contingencies. The protocol or care process that results is, at worst, completely unworkable, or, at best, used by only a portion of the clinical staff, never spread to others, and has little ability to be sustained over time. With this type of experience, most clinicians and improvement staff have concluded that standardization of clinical processes is almost impossible.

The fault lies in the methodology of development and implementation, however, not in the fundamental concept of standardization. Successful implementation of a standardized process demands and expects local customization. This means that a given standard or protocol is essentially never "finished," but is always in a state of adjustment as providers find better ways to provide care. Following are some recommended steps to standardize a process:

- Step 1. Describe the current and ideal process. By observation, identification of problems, and drilling down for root causes of process failures, understand how the current process works. Describe the ideal process for management of the condition, using evidence from the literature, knowledge of the local environment, and any available local data.

- Step 2. Define and implement a practical measurement strategy. The measurement should be practical both for short-term testing and longer-term outcomes.

- Step 3. Write the protocol or care process. The first draft of the protocol or care process should be written by several of the pertinent experts, taking a minimum of time, and utilizing out-of-organization examples of protocols, if necessary, just to get a start. The initial protocol or care process should be reflective of the few experts who will be willing to try the first version of the protocol on several patients within the next day or so. The protocol should be written in such a way that changes to the protocol or care process can be made within minutes. The goal for most organizations should be to include as few items as possible combined with good evidence.

• Step 4. Send out an early draft. Stakeholders should be encouraged to comment with short turnaround time limits to begin the buy-in process and improve the safety and robustness of the protocol.

• Step 5. Test an early draft of the protocol. The early draft of the protocol should be tested with a few patients. Immediately after these patients have been tested, the authors of the protocol should huddle with nurses and other staff who will be using the protocol to discuss what worked well and what needs to be changed. The information should immediately be incorporated into the protocol for the next series of tests.

• Step 6. Seek additional input from other interested participants. The initially tested and modified protocol should now be recommunicated with all other clinicians and staff who will eventually use the protocol, and further input requested. The input should then be used to remodel the protocol. The remodeled protocol should be tested and continually remodified as needed.

• Step 7. Set expectations on use of the protocol. Expect either that the protocol will actually be used, or that the reason for opting out is communicated to the development team whenever a clinician decides not to use the protocol. This feedback information is crucial for remodeling and improving the protocol as necessary.

• Step 8. Assign a process or protocol owner. The ability to sustain a protocol is dependent on an owner. The owner of a protocol has several responsibilities, including being aware of any new literature that would impact the protocol, having available the compliance data regarding the use of the protocol, and having basic data regarding the reasons why the protocol is not being used, if applicable. No changes can be made to the protocol without consent and delegation of those changes from the process owner.

• Step 9. Remodel the protocol. Changes should be made to the protocol based on identified problems with the protocol or issues relating to the nonuse of the protocol. Modifications and improvements of the protocol should be

an ongoing and continuous process. In essence, no protocol should ever be finished. The protocol should always be in the design mode.

Initial standardization of a care process will never be perfect, and the designers should expect failures. If an attempt is made in the initial design to deal with any and all probabilities that engage the clinical process, the initial protocol will become far too complicated. A complicated design is much more difficult to understand by the frontline staff that need to implement the protocol.

When the standardization process is inclusive and everyone has input, then acceptance and utilization increase. The process of testing, measuring, and improving the protocol also creates agreement between clinicians and provides certainty that the protocol is an improvement in care delivery.

As previously mentioned, the goal of step 1 is to achieve 80%–90% reliability. Your organization should have measures in place to gauge the reliability of the process. If it is not achieving 80%–90% reliability, then it should be redesigned and reworked to achieve the target reliability goal.

Step 2: Identification and Mitigation

Step 2 involves designing and implementing a process that "catches" those times when the step 1 process doesn't work and addressing the failures. Also known as the identification and mitigation step, it is critical to improving the reliability of a process. The second step allows for a less than perfect design in the standardization step, so you do not have to plan for every possible contingency in the first tier. For example, let's assume your organization's primary, standardized process for giving patients a pneumococcal vaccine is the nurse asking the patient during the final meeting before discharge whether he or she needs a pneumococcal vaccine and providing it when necessary. And let's assume that process works 80% of the time. Then to catch the 20% of patients not caught by the primary process you might implement a process in which visiting nurses who see the patient after discharge ask about the pneumococcal vaccine.

The goal of the second step is to catch 80% of the failures not caught in the primary process. Ultimately, if your second-step process catches 80% of the errors of the first-step process, your total system process will achieve 96% reliability.

Sidebar 4-1. Human Factors Engineering Strategies

Human factors engineering strategies to use in redesigning processes include the following:

- Avoid reliance on memory. This may involve designing processes to involve checklists, forced reminders, mnemonic devices, and so forth.

- Use constraints/forcing functions. These are functions that make it easy to do the right thing and hard to do the wrong thing. For example, in a computerized prescriber order entry system a constraint may be a notice that pops up on-screen when you enter an incorrect dose of medication. A forcing function in such a system may not allow you to proceed to the next screen without first performing a certain task, such as verifying allergies.

- Use protocols and checklists to generate standard care and, as previously mentioned, ensure that a procedure is performed consistently because the checklist detects inadvertent omission without relying on human memory.

- Decrease "look-alikes" and "sound-alikes." When two things look alike, it is easy to mistake one for another. Consider the soda aisle of a grocery store. The brand name cola is often placed next to a generic that has the same color label and font style. The differences between the labels are subtle, and when consumers are distracted or in a hurry, they may mistake one for the other. The same applies in health care with medications, supplies, equipment, and so forth. By reducing look-alikes, organizations can ensure that individuals will correctly identify the right product even when in a hurry, distracted, fatigued, or stressed. Within its National Patient Safety Goals, The Joint Commission requires organizations to limit look-alike medications to improve the reliability of medication delivery. In addition, The Joint Commission requires organizations to label all medications, medication containers (for example, syringes, medicine cups, basins), or other solutions on and off the sterile field to ensure accurate identification of medication and prevent medication error.

- Reduce the number of handoffs. The more times a patient is handed off to another provider, the more times important information about that patient can be lost. By limiting handoffs, you can limit the opportunity for error. Whenever handoffs are necessary, they should be structured so that consistent and comprehensive communication takes place every time. More about communication during handoffs can be found in Chapter 6.

- Automate carefully. As discussed in Chapter 10, technology can help streamline and standardize processes; however, it can also be a double-edged sword. Before implementing automation and technology, make sure that the process you are automating is effective, that the technology will ensure the consistent functioning of the process, and that the technology will not lead to workarounds or other new sources of error. Limited pilot projects that are carefully tracked can prevent major technology-induced problems.

- Take advantage of habits and patterns. If a new process works within the current habits and patterns of the participants in the process, they are more likely to embrace the new process and follow it. People inherently do not like change, so if a process can use components of an existing process it can prove to be more beneficial.

The second step is really all about using human factors in a design to identify defects. (*See* Sidebar 4-1, above.) A frequent approach is to use redundancy. Redundancies need to be carefully considered because they do represent a form of "waste" and should not be a complete re-audit. In general, they need to be independent of the original process used in the first step.

Within the second step you must set up a measurement tool to determine how often the step 2 process catches an error. A process rarely used will erode over time and not be dependable. A process used too frequently suggests a poorly designed first-tier standardization step and warrants some basic redesign.

Step 3: Failure Identification and Improvement

The effort in the third design step consists of two components. The first is the careful identification of failures that allow 5% of patients to be missed by the system as designed so far. The second is the careful creation of a direct link between these defects and a proposed redesign. All designs need a measurement of defects. Understanding why initial designs fail, and using the information about failures to redesign, is an essential part of reliability work. These defects provide the learning necessary to take the design to the desired level of reliability. The causes of the observed defects need to be prioritized, and then the highest-priority defects used for redesigning either the first or second tier. For this to occur, both components of the third tier need to be in place. The feedback loop to the design should be deliberate and swift to ensure rapid redesign.

By measuring a series of "small tests of change" and measuring their impact, a team can rapidly move from the "setup" phase of reliable design, all the way through step 3. After the process is part of routine operations and spread as

Figure 4-2. Reliable Design Checklist

Step 1: Standardization, Simplification, and Intent
Standardization and simplification of process
- "What" should be done? based on good medical evidence
- "How" can that be done? does not need medical evidence but systems knowledge

Ensure that each step is necessary: reducing # of steps can reduce error.
Initial standardized protocols: small-time investment by experts.
Customization initially: required and encouraged.
Changes are possible when generally accepted, but monitored.
Design the process so you can learn from each defect.
Leadership must drive expectation of standardization.
Model shifts from "opt in" to "opt out."
Designated process owner
Reach 80%–90% compliance before next step.

Step 2: Apply Controls
Decision aids and reminders built into the system
- Use hierarchy of controls (mitigate–facilitate–eliminate)

Teamwork and communication tools used
Desired action is the default (based on evidence).
Building process into scheduled steps (for example, daily rounds)
Take advantage of habits and patterns (for example, change-of-shift report).
Aim is to reach 90% to 95% before next step is designed.

Step 3: Identification and Mitigation
Through the use of redundancies, failures that occur are identified and mitigated (before they cause harm) to go as far beyond 95% reliability as feasible.
Make sure you have a way to count how many times the redundancy is needed to stop harm (For example, if needed more than 5%–10% of time, revisit design).

Ongoing process improvement
Measure critical *failures.*
If you are going to pursue, this is where "customization" occurs—that is, a different process may be needed for outliers.
This should be used to redesign the process when appropriate (> 10% failure).

This figure offers a checklist that organizations can use to help navigate the reliable design process.

Source: Doug Bonacum, Kaiser Permanente. Used with permission.

appropriate, future failures can be studied, and redesign implemented if it makes sense from a cost/benefit perspective.

ADDRESSING THE CULTURAL ASPECTS OF RELIABILITY

As mentioned in Chapter 1, designing reliable processes is only one step in becoming a high-reliability organization. Your organization must address the cultural piece as well. A clear example of the need to address culture when designing for reliability is the often doubted efficacy of bar coding, a technology that from an engineering and reliable process perspective is a "no brainer." The issue with bar coding in many organizations however, may be more about the organization's culture, patient safety values, how the technology is socialized in the organization, and how leaders listen and respond to staff members who are having trouble using it safely.

Likewise, the ongoing debate about the efficacy of rapid response teams (*see* Chapter 13 on pages 122–124) appears to be one grounded in culture as well. If the concept of the rapid response team is not appropriately introduced in an organization, if the culture is not "just" nor one where it's safe to speak up, and if the organization doesn't place a high value on continuous learning from both the appropriate use and failure to use the system, rapid response teams might be another great safety idea that falls short in execution.

Ensuring effective teamwork and communication, developing a just culture and accountability system, and examining mistakes in order to learn from them are just some of the concepts that must be in place to achieve a culture of reliability. Another piece is to develop an organizational intolerance for ambiguity and workarounds. In his article, "Fixing Health Care from the Inside, Today" author Steven Spear compares and contrasts the U.S. health care system with the Toyota Production System,[4] noting that health care workers work around ambiguities, meeting patients' immediate needs but not resolving the ambiguities themselves. As a result, people confront the same problem, every day, for years, manifested as inefficiencies and irritations—and, occasionally, as catastrophes. Unless everyone is completely clear about the tasks that must be done, exactly who should be doing them, and just how they should be performed, Spear notes, the potential for error will always be high.

REFERENCES

1. Berwick D., Nolan T.: High reliability health care. Paper presented at the Institute for Healthcare Improvement's 15th Annual Forum on Quality Improvement in Health Care, New Orleans, Dec. 2003.

2. McGlynn E.A., et al.: The quality of health care delivered to adults in the United States. *N Eng J Med* 48:2635–2645, 2003.

3. Reinertsen J.L.: Zen and the art of physician autonomy maintenance. *Ann Intern Med* 138:992–995, Jun. 17, 2003.

4. Spear S.J.: Fixing healthcare from the inside: Teaching residents to heal broken delivery processes as they heal sick patients. *Acad Med* 81(suppl.):S144, 2006.

Chapter Five

SYSTEMATIC FLOW
OF INFORMATION

Allan Frankel and *Sarah Grillo*

One of the primary tenets of this book is that leaders should foster an environment in which errors, near misses, risks, and problems are discussed openly and honestly, and then acted upon. To do this, organizations must have a systematic flow of information from frontline staff to organization leadership and back again. This helps ensure a reliable system in which problems and risks are consistently identified; identified issues are analyzed; staff concerns are responded to; and risks are addressed in such a way that experience facilitates prevention, identification, or mitigation of future errors. An organization that has a systematic flow of information takes a significant step toward high reliability and enhances its patient safety and performance.

There are some critical elements involved in systemizing the flow of information, including the following:

• Easy-to-use methods of capturing information about problems or issues

• Leadership support of and active participation in these methods

• A consistently reinforced message to staff that speaking up or reporting concerns and events is an esteemed action that may be done safely. A systematic flow of information is predicated on a robust, easily understandable accountability system in which staff members know when they will be held accountable for safety and reliability failures and when the organization will hold accountable the systems that support the provision of health care in the organization. As discussed in Chapter 3, organizations must assess accountability consistently to ensure that staff knows how the organization will respond to problems or errors.

• A mechanism for organizing and ranking the information collected. Most organizations don't have the time and funds to fix every problem that staff members encounter. By prioritizing, organizations can determine, out of the 100 problems identified, which 5 are the most important to fix right away. One effective method for ranking information is to consider the severity of the issue and multiply it by how many times that issue occurs. Issues that are high severity and high frequency should go to the top of the list.[1] Organizations may also consider fixing issues that are low severity but high frequency, as these are the little irritations that staff faces every day. High-severity, low-frequency events may also be important to address depending on the nature of the problem and the likelihood of the frequency.

• An owner for the information gathering, analysis, and response process. Recently, organizations are combining quality and safety and risk departments to support this effort.

• Prompt acknowledgement of reports. Even if you cannot fix a problem right away, it is important to acknowledge the report and outline what the next steps are in addressing it.

• Regular and comprehensive communication about issue resolution. When an issue is resolved, you must communicate to everyone about the nature of the problem and how it got fixed. It's important for staff members to see action as a result of their speaking up or reporting. If they believe that they do so and nothing is done about it, they will stop reporting. Establishing a systematic flow of information does not have to be hard. Some effective tools that can help you do this include the following:

—Executive WalkRounds™
—Glitch Book
—Spontaneous Reporting System

—Review of failures identified through routine record review, deaths, severe adverse events, and so forth

EXECUTIVE WALKROUNDS™

Executive WalkRounds™ are a stimulated information-gathering tool in which management and front line staff engage in a structured, two-way conversation about safety, and data from that conversation are captured, analyzed, prioritized, and addressed.[2] On the whole, the WalkRounds process is designed to do the following:

• Show senior leaders that are promoting patient safety efforts.

• Hear the concerns of frontline providers. Through WalkRounds, leaders get to directly interact with staff, learn the unfiltered truth about issues, and directly influence the tone of the culture.

• Increase mutual understanding between senior leaders and frontline staff about patient safety issues.

• Support appropriate accountability.

• Foster a culture of teamwork and continuous learning.

• Allocate resources to areas of greatest risk.

How To Conduct WalkRounds[3]

The WalkRounds process is fairly straightforward and includes the following seven steps:

1. Preparation. This step involves garnering commitment and regular participation by leadership, securing dedicated resources from quality and safety departments, and clearly defining the process, scheduling, and feedback mechanisms for the rest of the organization.

2. Scheduling. To be effective, organizations should consider setting WalkRounds months in advance and accommodate schedules of executive team members, supporting patient safety staff, and other participants. Canceling these scheduled rounds should be strongly discouraged, with agreement that rather than ever canceling, leaders commit to rescheduling within a short time frame.

3. Conducting WalkRounds. A first step is to decide where to conduct the sessions. WalkRounds take about an hour to complete and can occur at any site in the organization where employees or clinicians are directly involved in patient care or support the process, including all hospital floors, radiology, emergency rooms, pharmacies, ambulatory settings, and outpatient offices. WalkRounds have also been done in the hospital billing office, central sterilization units, transportation departments, and on floors dedicated to hospital information technology systems. When choosing a site, you may want to consider starting with those units in which the safety climate score—of the safety culture assessment survey discussed in Chapter 2—is less than 60. This indicates an area in which a strong rapport between leadership and frontline staff could be very beneficial.

When conducting the WalkRounds, you may hold the discussion on the floor or department in an open area to increase visibility or, at the discretion of the leaders or department, in a back room or empty patient room. There are advantages to each of these modes. If the discussion is held in the nursing station, staff working on the unit can observe the group in conversation and learn about the WalkRounds. The WalkRounds should be open for anyone to participate; hospitals that conduct the WalkRounds in an open area can stop clinicians who pass by and ask them to participate. If WalkRounds are conducted in a back room, such as a coffee lounge, participants are less likely to be pulled away for clinical issues. Interestingly, neither location seems detrimental to the candor of the conversation, and both modes are able to elicit comments on complex issues related to patient care and adverse events.

Sessions should include an opening statement (see Sidebar 5-1 on page 41), and leaders should ask some detailed questions to prompt discussion. Questions may include the following:

• "What did we do that harmed a patient?"

• "How will we harm the next patient?"

• "What doesn't work well?"

• "What are you worried might happen that could hurt a patient?"

• "Do some ethnic groups get better care here than others?"

• "Do we disclose all that we reasonably should to patients, including mistakes and potential mistakes?"

• "How well does teamwork occur on this unit?"

These, and questions like these, will elicit different responses. For example, a night nurse might report that, "At 5 A.M., an anticoagulated patient fell out of bed and hit her head and started bleeding. I paged four different physicians before I found the on-call physician. The patient lost a unit of blood." Other comments from employees may range from, "The new bar-coding scanners won't accurately scan the IV bags again." to "The IV pole wheels were sticking. The patient tripped and cut her knee as a result. Her IV infiltrated at the same time."

The patient safety officer plays a critical role during the WalkRounds. He or she should ensure that only one conversation is conducted at any one time and help encourage quieter individuals to speak up. The senior leader can act as moderator if skilled and interested, but the patient safety officer should be responsible for, and capable of, making the rounds productive, inclusive, and focused.

Within the WalkRounds, all participants should be encouraged to give feedback. To ensure that all individuals are able to voice their concerns and that more reserved individuals will have an opportunity to speak, the patient safety officer or senior leader might consider asking the most junior individuals specifically about their concerns or take turns asking each individual in the group to comment on the topic being discussed.

During the WalkRound, the scribe should be taking notes. The scribe is one of, if not the most, critical participants in the WalkRounds process. It is his or her job to document information about what was said, who said it, and what the response was. Scribes in organizations performing WalkRounds have ranged from research assistants to the senior administrative assistant of the quality and safety department. Though a pad of paper will suffice for taking notes, many organizations use tabular forms that facilitate real-time sorting of concerns and start the process of distinguishing adverse events from their contributing factors. These forms should include the following fields:

- Date of WalkRound
- Location (unit, floor, and, if applicable, facility)
- Names of executives present
- Names of patient safety staff present
- For each comment, name of person speaking
- Concerns elicited from the unit on previous WalkRounds
  - When elicited, contributing factors to concerns
  - Status of any prior concerns

When the WalkRound has finished, the scribe will enter data collected into the database for further analysis.

After WalkRounds conclude, the executive team should immediately debrief on site (*see* information on debriefing in Chapter 6), assign urgent action items if needed, and together compare the scribe notes with the team's under-

---

Sidebar 5-1. Sample Open and Closing Statements

Although opening statements will vary among different organizations, following are a sample opening and closing statement used successfully across some organizations who conduct Executive WalkRounds™.

Opening Statement

"We are moving as an organization to open communication and a just culture environment because we believe that doing so will make your work environment safer for you and your patients. The discussion we are interested in having with you is confidential and purely for patient safety and improvement. We are interested in focusing on the systems you work in each day rather than on blaming specific individuals. The questions we might ask you will tend to be general ones, and you might consider how these questions might apply in your work areas in regards to medication errors, communication or teamwork problems, distractions, inefficiencies, problems with protocols, etc. We are happy to discuss any issues of concern to you. Our goal is to take what we learn in these conversations and use them to improve your work environment and our overall delivery of care."

Closing Statement

"We appreciate the time and effort you put into taking care of patients and making their experience in our organization remarkable. Our job is to take the information you have given us, analyze it carefully, figure out what actions we might take to fix problems, assign those responsibilities to individuals, and hold their feet to the fire until the problems are solved. We promise to let you know how we're doing and we will come back and elicit your opinion. We will work on the information you have given us. In return we would like you to tell two other people you work with about the concepts we have discussed in this conversation. As you see or think of other adverse events or are concerned about potential harm to a patient please report it by _____ (fill in the mechanism to be used in particular organization). Near misses and adverse events are windows that we can all use to improve the safety of care we deliver. We can only address the issues if we know and talk about them openly."

Source: Allan Frankel. Used with permission.

---

standing of the issues. The scribe should add to his or her notes any other insights generated during this discussion. The group should discuss what went well, what went poorly, and what was learned, and possibly begin prioritizing important issues and potential improvements.

4. **Tracking.** To effectively track information gleaned during the Executive WalkRounds process, organizations should set up a robust system for tracking and ranking collected data, such as an interactive database that allows for sorting and prioritizing. (*See* Sidebar 5-2, right.) Using a database, organizations can accomplish the following:

- Track names of individuals who participate in each WalkRound.

- Note location, time, and date of each round.

- Record comments given and hazards identified during the rounds.

- Identify the contributing factors.

- Develop actions to address the issues.

- Link specific comments with the individuals who initially discussed them.

- Link comments with those charged to fix them.

Within the tracking system, it may be beneficial to have a systemized way of ranking issues. This may involve the previously mentioned severity $\times$ frequency approach or other method.

Information from the WalkRounds process should be integrated with other data, including reporting system, root cause analyses, surveillance, and audit data. The patient safety team is typically responsible for synthesizing data, integrating with other organizational data, and helping with prioritization. This involves categorizing WalkRounds comments, determining action items, presenting information to the multidisciplinary group, and tracking progress on any initiatives.

5. **Reporting.** After information has been entered and analyzed, organizations should share data with a multidisciplinary committee so that action items may be assigned to management personnel. Often the patient safety committee is the designated committee to receive WalkRounds information. Although this is often appropriate, the data collected from WalkRounds are frequently broader than "safety" alone and some link to an administrative and clinical operations group is required. From there, different committee members can take ownership of different projects or initiatives.

6. **Feedback.** A critical element to the WalkRounds process is a clearly delineated and formal structure for feedback to frontline providers who participate in WalkRounds, and to executive boards about findings and actions taken to address issues brought up in WalkRounds. By using formal

---

Sidebar 5-2. Using a Database to Track Information

Brigham and Women's Hospital in Boston has been using WalkRounds™ to identify patient safety issues for many years. To help sort, track, and analyze data collected during the WalkRounds, the team designed an Access database, which has been refined over a seven-year period and effectively used by other hospitals around the country. Demographic information can be entered into the database and correlated with events elicited during each WalkRound. Built into the database are templates for reports that can be structured in a manner useful for executive leadership or with greater detail for specific departments or managers. (*See* Figure 5-1 on page 43.)

The database tracks information from the time it is elicited during WalkRounds through the assignment of contributing factors,[4] the identification of actions to be taken, notation for when action is taken, responsibility for follow-up, and final disposition. An action is deemed complete (problem resolved) or closed (addressed as fully as possible) only when it is communicated back to the front line and more specifically to the individual(s) who raised the issue during WalkRounds.

---

methods of feedback, your organization can ensure the appropriate buy-in from all levels in the organization, foster commitment to the WalkRounds process, and facilitate planning, prioritization, and assignment of action items.

When communicating to the frontline staff, organizations should communicate that staff members' comments are valued and will lead to change in care delivery. When you are just starting to implement WalkRounds, staff may be hesitant to report issues or may believe that the information reported is insubstantial or awkward. After the frontline providers and managers realize the benefits to be accrued—that improvements actually occur—the conversations become more open and robust. There are many effective ways to communicate with staff, including the following:

- Memos or e-mails to individual providers. Within such notes, you can thank staff for joining in the conversation, identify the major topics discussed, and review those slated for further analysis and action.

- Newsletter articles

- Periodic data summaries to managers for dissemination to staff

- Town hall meetings with executives to highlight accomplishments

Figure 5-1. WalkRounds™ Database

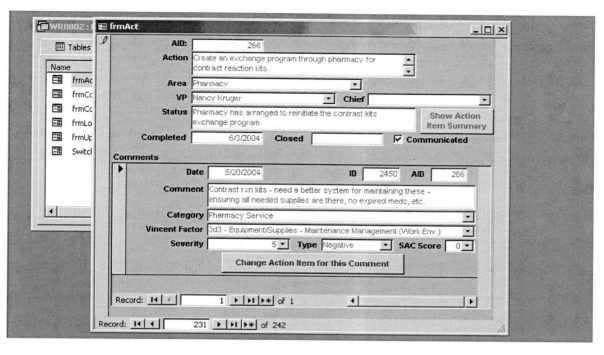

This figure shows a snapshot of the Executive WalkRounds database used by Brigham and Women's Hospital in Boston.

Source: Brigham and Women's Hospital, Boston. Used with permission.

• Dashboards that communicate the status of critical issues

Feedback should occur promptly. Even if action is delayed, the staff person should receive feedback on what is being done to address his or her issue. Organizations should deliver feedback in multiple and redundant ways to make sure the information is clearly visible, received, and understood by all.

Communication with executive boards can take the form of monthly reports to senior and physician leaders, quarterly reports to patient safety/quality committees, and biannual reports to boards.

7. Measurement. It is important to evaluate whether WalkRounds are effective in improving the organization's culture. As discussed in Chapter 2, a number of validated surveys are available to quantify caregivers' attitudes and perceptions of their working environments. WalkRounds have been directly linked with improvements in cultural perceptions and attitudes about teamwork, perceptions of management, willingness to speak up, and the overall safety of the working environment.[5,6]

Success Is Dependent on Senior Leadership

For WalkRounds to be successful, there must be an overt commitment from senior leadership. Such a commitment involves more than just an agreement to join meetings held by patient safety personnel or an individual department head. The decision is a team and process commitment, and includes the following actions:

• Demonstrate leadership and involvement in the actual WalkRounds sessions—this responsibility is first and foremost.

• Help make connections between problems, issues, and suggested changes.

• Ensure follow-through on issues at the executive level. Many issues will rise to the operating committee and likely become part of capital appropriations discussions.

• Demonstrate organizational commitment to this process and to patient safety.

• Chair monthly meetings of a multidisciplinary committee to review and act on data gathered during the rounds.

• Participate in feedback to employees and departments.

In short, WalkRounds should be more than an opportunity for hospital leaders to take the floor and expound on their feelings or pet projects, listen and shake hands, or address randomly noted items written on a 3 × 5 card. The substance of WalkRounds comes from an effective dialogue among all participants. The degree of personal satisfaction for each individual who participates will be determined by how effectively the backroom efforts after WalkRounds are brought to fruition. Tracking data carefully and ensuring that follow-up actions are taken—in essence, great leadership—will determine how interesting and effective the WalkRounds become.[3]

Realistically, some hospital leaders will have the personality and skill set to make WalkRounds successful. Others will not. Leaders can learn the skills necessary to perform good WalkRounds, and it is the responsibility of good organizations to equip their leaders with the skills to succeed in the WalkRounds process.

Before engaging in the WalkRounds process, organizations should evaluate their leaders. One evaluation of leadership that might be useful is whether leaders accurately evaluate the state of affairs in their organizations or domains of responsibility. Leaders tend to fit into three categories: those who are overly optimistic compared to the assessments of their frontline providers, those who are overly pessimistic about the state of affairs in their domains of responsibility compared to the frontline providers who work in those units, and those whose perceptions are similar to those of the frontline providers. The ideal leader falls into the third category. Leadership perceptions can be evaluated using attitudinal surveys and through focused interviews.

WalkRounds will be most successful in those organizations that are willing to assess their leaders and choose only those with suitable personalities and perspectives to lead WalkRounds. In addition, successful organizations will assess their units using attitudinal surveys to identify those units most in need of leadership engagement and where attitudes toward safety, teamwork, and management are poor. This combination of thoughtful framing of both leaders and units prior to or as the WalkRounds process begins is likely to yield the best results for the significant effort required to implement and sustain a WalkRounds program.

GLITCH BOOK

The glitch book is a tool that is located at the point of care

and offers frontline providers a chance to immediately and quickly document problems, issues, or concerns that require attention. The name "glitch" comes from work done by Paul Uhlig and Jeff Brown to improve cardiac surgery through multidisciplinary teamwork[7] and stands for Glimmers of Little Information that Catch Harm. The "book" may take the form of a notebook with designated areas in which to document concerns or may work better in an easily accessible electronic format. Either way, the glitch books offers frontline staff the opportunity to share problems while they are fresh in the mind. For example, if a surgeon and nurse in the operating room notice that a piece of equipment is not working correctly, they can immediately go to the glitch book and enter information about that piece of equipment for further attention.

For the glitch book concept to work, the following elements must be present:

• It must be easily accessible and easy to use. Often, providers just write down the description of a problem within the glitch book along with the date and time of the entry and the provider name.

• It must be regularly reviewed by unit leaders, quality leaders, or other designated individuals. In the case of an office-based practice, the physician owner of the practice may review the glitch book. Within this review, leaders should ask the following questions:

—How problematic are the concerns?

—What are the contributing factors causing them?

—What are the actions that might be taken to fix the concerns?

—Who is accountable for taking those actions?

—After action is taken, who will provide feedback to people who put information in the glitch book?

• It must have an owner. This individual or group is responsible not only for regularly reviewing the glitch book but also making sure that issues are addressed in an appropriate and timely manner.

• Issues must be addressed 100% of the time, meaning that every comment is acted upon, or feedback is given to the individuals who raised the concern about why the problem will not be addressed. Information within the glitch book will divide into the following categories:

—Problems that can be fixed now on the unit, such as if patients are slipping on shower floors, nonslip carpeting or material can be placed onto the shower floors.

—Problems that represent an issue between units, such as if material management is supplying intravenous bags to the supply closet, but not effectively monitoring the use and par levels of the items despite repeated requests to do so. In this case unit leaders will need to figure how to fix the problem together and who is going to own it. If one unit doesn't want to be involved in fixing the problem, then information needs to be fed back to the WalkRounds process to facilitate the two units to work together.

—Problems that are more global in nature. In this case, information should be fed back up to the Executive WalkRounds process. An example of a problem that is bigger than a unit problem is the computerized prescriber order entry system or a bar-coding system that is used organizationwide and in which the batteries in the bar coding devices have an unacceptable failure rate.

Whatever type of problem, the organization must commit to addressing it—whether by fixing it immediately or referring it to the quality department for review. As with other types of reporting systems, organizations should provide feedback to individuals who report issues as to what is being done about the issue, even if the "what is being done" is a discussion where the conclusion is to not take action.

Relationship Between WalkRounds and Glitch Book

While WalkRounds is a mechanism for engaging senior leadership in safety, the glitch book relies on the participation of frontline staff and takes a unit-level approach to gathering information. Because information gathered in the glitch book is often written as free text and because, in theory, every unit has a glitch book, information from the glitch book can be very difficult, if not impossible, to aggregate across multiples units. However, organizations should have a mechanism to share information between the glitch book and the WalkRounds process. For example, when a unit-level issue is discovered in the Executive WalkRounds, there should be a mechanism by which information about the issue is communicated to the group or individual that "owns" the unit glitch book. As previously mentioned, when a glitch book reveals an organizationwide issue, there should be a mechanism by which information is fed to senior leadership who are reviewing, analyzing, and prioritizing information at the global level.

WalkRounds and glitch books are examples of continuous learning cycles that exist concurrently at the organization and unit level. You may envision them as parts of a large circle linked to many smaller overlapping circles, all steadily turning, with occasional pieces moving from one circle to another in a consistently complex pattern but characterized by smooth transitions, one and all.

SPONTANEOUS REPORTING SYSTEM

A spontaneous reporting system is one in which any individual in the hospital—clinician, employee, volunteer, patient, or family member—can report an issue, concern, or problem. Such a system should be designed to capture all issues from all persons whether employed or independent—both global and unit specific—in an organization. If all groups reported then when aggregated, information from a spontaneous reporting system would give a comprehensive picture of risk in the organization. In reality in health care, reporting systems tend to be utilized preferentially by some disciplines such as nursing, and very little by others, such as physicians. The data generated by analysis of these reporting systems become just one lens on the organization. Organizations should consider how representative reported data are by evaluating the reporters and comparing the data with that from other safety-related organizational databases, such as risk management files and the WalkRounds and glitch book collections.

Ideally, a spontaneous reporting system captures and analyzes information in such a way that problems missed elsewhere are captured here. One way of thinking of it is that a spontaneous reporting system ensures reliability in the problem identification process by capturing information the Executive WalkRounds and glitch book may miss. For example, if two units are experiencing a similar problem with the pharmacy, such as trouble receiving medications in a timely manner, and they both report the problem in their glitch book, because the glitch book is a more unit-based data collection tool and is very difficult to aggregate across units, leaders may miss the fact that the same issue is occurring in two different units. A spontaneous reporting system would catch both those reports and clearly make the link between the two.

Ideally, information gathered in a spontaneous reporting system goes directly to the patient safety office. The patient safety officer owns the reporting system and is responsible for regularly reviewing data within the system, analyzing it, and prioritizing it for improvement. Because of his or her involvement with other reporting systems, the patient safety officer and/or the quality assurance department is in the unique position to see a more global perspective on issues revealed by the system.

There are a variety of mechanisms for spontaneous reporting, including via telephone, a Web-based form, an e-mail, a paper form, and so forth. Of all the mechanisms, the electronic formats may be the most helpful because of the speed of reporting and ease of analysis.

There are some challenges to a spontaneous reporting system. If it is structured so that individuals report using free text, information from the spontaneous reporting system may be difficult to aggregate, such as with the glitch book. However, if a form is developed with checkboxes that individuals can fill in, critical information may be lost if a prompt is not present on the form. In addition, if the form has many different fields to complete, it may be time-consuming and end up being a deterrent for reporting. Consequently, spontaneous reporting systems must balance between a format that is easy for staff to use and one that is easy for the patient safety office to analyze.

Another issue associated with the spontaneous reporting system is the level of anonymity of the reporters. If you make such a system anonymous, then people will feel more free to report issues, concerns, and events. However, problems may arise when you are unable to gain more information if the initial report is incomplete. Ideally, your organization will establish an environment in which frontline providers believe that their comments are held in high enough regard; that positive actions are taken on reported information; that there is a high enough level of reasonable accountability; that they know they won't be blamed for a system error; and that regular reporting will help improve the organization and the safety of patients. In other words, a just culture with appropriate accountability is the environment in which a sponta- neous reporting system becomes the most useful.

PATIENT SAFETY OFFICERS MUST LOOK AT THE BIG PICTURE

Executive WalkRounds, glitch books, and spontaneous reporting systems are only a few ways to identify risk in an organization. Other methods include the following:

1. Risk management incident reports

2. Malpractice reports

3. Customer complaints

4. Trigger tools (*See* Sidebar 5-3, below.)

The data in each of these are fodder for continuous learning cycles.

The tricky thing with all these different sources of information is that often different people in the health care organization see different pieces of the pie, so no one gets an entire picture of incidents in the organization. Your organization must commit to designating responsibility to one individual or department to look at the big picture and see where improvement opportunities lie. In most cases, that individual would be the patient safety officer and the department under his or her watch, although in some organizations clinically oriented risk managers and quality leaders hold the right position.

The name of this game is cyclic continuous learning in which action bolsters the desire of health care workers to

---

Sidebar 5-3. IHI Global Trigger Tool[8]

The use of "triggers," or clues to identify adverse events (AEs) that cause harm to patients is an effective method for measuring the overall level of harm from medical care in a health care organization. Institute for Healthcare Improvement (IHI) has created the following trigger tools, which provide an easy-to-use method for accurately identifying AEs and measuring the rate of AEs over time. The following tools provide an organizationwide measure that can be reported to leadership and is designed for use with the records of adult inpatients in acute care:

- IHI Global Trigger Tool for Measuring Inpatient Adverse Events
- Trigger Tool for Measuring Adverse Drug Events
- Surgical Trigger Tool for Measuring Perioperative Adverse Events
- Intensive Care Unit Adverse Event Trigger Tool
- Trigger Tool for Measuring Adverse Events in the Neonatal Intensive Care Unit
- Outpatient Adverse Event Trigger Tool

Tracking AEs over time is a useful way to tell if changes being made are improving the safety of the care processes. With all Trigger Tools, data should always be tracked over time and categorized for review, such as in a histogram. This may identify further focus areas for work. Intensive review using a subset of triggers can be very helpful, such as anticoagulant-related harm in medications, and may be used for focused improvement efforts.

participate, speak up, and report. By looking at all the variety of information sources, the patient safety officer can get a better picture of what's going on in the organization safety-wise. He or she can identify critical areas that need leadership involvement and unit-level issues that need to be addressed. He or she can help smooth the flow of information and ensure that issues are consistently identified, prioritized, and addressed.

REFERENCES

1. Bagian J.P., et al.: The Veterans Affairs root cause analysis system in action. *Jt Comm J Qual Improv* 28:531–545, 2002.

2. Frankel A., et al.: Patient safety leadership WalkRounds™. *Jt Comm J Qual Saf* 29:16–26, 2003.

3. Frankel A., Grillo S., Pittman M.: *Patient Safety Leadership WalkRounds™ Guide.* Cambridge, MA: Institute for Healthcare Improvement, 2004.

4. Vincent C.: Understanding and responding to adverse events. *N Engl J Med* 348:1051, Mar. 13, 2003.

5. Frankel A., et al.: Revealing and resolving patient safety defects: The impact of Leadership WalkRounds™ on frontline caregiver assessments of patient safety, *Health Serv Res* Jul. 29, 2008.

6. Thomas E.J., et al.: The effect of executive WalkRounds™ on nurse safety climate attitudes: A randomized trial of clinical units. *BMC Health Serv Res* 5:28, Apr. 11, 2005.

7. Uhlig P.N., et al.: John M. Eisenberg Patient Safety Awards. System innovation: Concord Hospital. *Jt Comm J Qual Improv* 12:666–672, Dec. 2002.

8. Institute for Healthcare Improvement: *Trigger Tools.* http://www.ihi.org/IHI/Topics/PatientSafety/SafetyGeneral/Tools/Introto TriggerToolsforIdentifyingAEs.htm (accessed Jul. 1, 2008).

Chapter Six

EFFECTIVE TEAMWORK AND COMMUNICATION

Michael Leonard, Allan Frankel, and *Terri Simmonds*

Fundamentally, effective communication is the accurate exchange of information between two or more people. It can be formal or informal, brief or lengthy, detailed or vague. Failures in communication occur when the information exchange is not complete, effective, or appropriate. When such communication failures occur within the health care setting, the consequences can be severe. Treatments can be overlooked, diagnoses missed, risks not addressed, and patients hurt. In fact, the overwhelming majority of untoward events in medicine involve communication failures.

Common communication mishaps resulting in patient harm include the following:

• Providing care with incomplete or missing information

• Executing poor handoffs with relevant clinical data not clearly communicated

• Failing to confirm, or read back, information transmitted

• Failing to share and communicate known information, such as when a team member knows there is a problem, but is unable to speak up about it. For example, there are many documented cases of wrong-site surgery that show that someone in the room was aware the surgeon was operating on the incorrect site but was afraid to speak up about it.

• Assuming the expected outcome and safety of care. Consider the following example: *An obstetrician came into the hospital to be present during the labor of a close personal friend. The hospital's obstetrical nurses saw worrisome changes on the fetal tracing monitor outside at the desk, but did not intervene because the nurses assumed the physician saw the tracing and recognized its significance. The physician, involved in social conversation, was not aware of the abnormal fetal tracing.*

Creating an environment centered on effective communication offers several benefits, including the following:

• Contributes to the consistent delivery of high-quality, safe patient care

• Allows staff to learn from mistakes rather than placing individual blame—helping care providers understanding how they work together effectively in a very complex environment.

• Is essential in managing the complexity of patient care in a setting that often exceeds the capabilities of an individual clinician

• Ensures staff safety

• Enhances learning and opportunity for improvement

• Provides a more satisfying and rewarding work environment for staff

• Fosters an environment in which health care organizations can attract and retain critically important employees, such as nurses, pharmacists, and physicians

• Supports better interactions with patients and families, with higher patient satisfaction

WHY IS EFFECTIVE COMMUNICATION SO DIFFICULT IN HEALTH CARE?

Despite its importance, ineffective communication is a pervasive problem in health care organizations. There are many possible reasons for this, including the following:

• Leadership has not prioritized effective communication and teamwork within the organization. As discussed in Chapter 1, a high-performance culture based on structured and open communication cannot exist without visible and sustained leadership commitment. While it is easy for leaders to say "we must communicate better," to achieve such a culture leaders must be open and honest about errors, actively participate in initiatives to improve communication, incorporate effective communication into policies and procedures, specifically train professionals in better communication techniques, foster the creation and maintenance of teams, and hold everyone—including themselves—accountable for effective communication.

- Many health care professionals greatly value autonomy and have trouble understanding the inherent value in teamwork.[1] As previously discussed, health care professionals are trained to be individual experts who work hard to provide patient care.[2] The idea of working as a team, valuing multiple inputs, and solving problems collaboratively is not inherent in many providers' way of thinking. They also have not been trained to appreciate the value of effective leadership, including how "setting the stage" every time the team comes together not only to share information but also create an environment in which everyone knows the plan, feels valued, and has been invited to speak up and voice both suggestions and concerns. Systematically showing providers the value of working collaboratively needs to be an organizational goal. The philosophy of "if we all just come together and do our jobs" greatly increases the risk of an adverse event when working in a complex environment full of surprises.

- Certain hierarchies are present within health care, and other types of organizations, that act as a barrier to effective communication.[3] Anytime a physician interacts with a nurse, a pharmacist, or other physicians, hierarchy and power distances exist. The perceived degree of hierarchy has a profound effect on the willingness of people to speak up, particularly to question a decision or identify a problem. Being at the top of the clinical hierarchy, physicians are typically less aware of the issue and the interpersonal dynamics that are created. Good leaders actively work to flatten hierarchy, minimize power distances, and consistently engage all team members.[4]

- The current, fragmented health care model reinforces and tolerates unstructured and often poor communication. For communication to be effective, organizational processes and systems must support and set the expectation of effective communication. For example, processes that include a repeat back to confirm information; include structured communication templates to ensure that all the information is present; and require all participants to be respected and encouraged to speak up foster effective communication. Conversely, processes that don't do this can actually reinforce poor communication and set up providers to fail.

- Failure of leadership to define and insist on an environment in which everyone is universally treated with respect. As noted in The Joint Commission *Sentinel Event Alert* in July 2008, abusive and disrespectful behavior is dangerous. According to the *Alert*, "Intimidating and disruptive behaviors can foster medical errors, contribute to poor patient satisfaction and to preventable adverse outcomes, increase the cost of care, and cause qualified clinicians, administrators and managers to seek new positions in more professional environments."[5] If someone at the bedside is hesitant to voice concern about a patient or call someone because "it wasn't too much fun the last time we interacted," then there is an unacceptable risk. As previously mentioned, clearly defining that abusive and disrespectful behavior is out of bounds and enforcing such a policy is critical to creating a high-performance culture that delivers safe care.

Most health care providers have not been systematically taught how to effectively communicate, particularly across health care disciplines. Medical, nursing, pharmacy, and other health care–related schools focus on clinical information and scientific knowledge, but do not have a central focus on how to effectively communicate, interact, and respond to peers, patients, and other providers. This lack of standardized approach means the different disciplines enter the clinical care environment with different styles, their own jargon, and little knowledge about the inherent value in standardized and clear communication.

For example, nurses have historically been taught to be narrative in their communication—"tell a story." This has been reinforced by the traditional nursing edict—"you don't make diagnoses." Physicians, on the other hand, are systematically trained to give "the 10-second version, the headlines." It is not that any one style is right or wrong, but they are different, and having a common and predictable structure for communication is extremely important to help navigate those differences. To compensate for health care providers' lack of communication skills, certain strategies and tools can enhance communication and foster teamwork. Such strategies and tools can be effectively applied in all clinical health care domains, inpatient and outpatient. Following is a discussion of some of these strategies and tools.

Set the Tone for Teamwork

Effective leaders set the stage for team interaction by creating and supporting an atmosphere in which people believe their input is valued and it is safe to ask questions, and they are comfortable speaking up if they don't understand or perceive a problem. Setting a positive tone for interaction can greatly promote cohesion and collaboration among individuals.[6] Conversely, a negative tone can inhibit communication and lead to error.

The team leader, consciously or unconsciously, sets the tone of collaboration very quickly—in about 5–10 seconds—through his or her verbal communication, body language, facial expressions, and attitude. As previously mentioned, most health care team leaders are unaware of the importance of actively setting a positive tone and the behaviors associated with such activity. In a recent observational study of 300 surgical cases, researchers noticed that surgeons were critical to setting the tone for team interaction. As they prepared for the next surgical case, operating room (OR) team members—nurses, technicians, and anesthesia providers—participated in active dialogue about the case, social issues, and so forth before the surgeon entered the room. Within 10 seconds of entering the room, the surgeon's behavior had a profound effect on the communication pattern in the room. If the surgeon engaged the team, set a positive tone, and shared the plan, all the communication continued. However, if he or she set a negative tone, all team communication was virtually eliminated.[7]

Consider this example. A surgeon runs into the room as the team is setting up for a hernia repair. He loudly proclaims, "I have a plane to catch in four hours, and we have a bunch of cases to do. Get on with it!" He is so fixated on getting the cases done and pushing the pace that he makes the incision on the wrong side, and the nurses watch—not knowing how to tell him or being willing to get in front of "the speeding train." Unfortunately, this story is true.

Most leaders set the stage for interactions informally or by default. A better idea is to actively set the stage with the message that "we're all contributing value to the care of this patient, this is a team sport, and we will work together in a respectful, open manner that encourages collaboration and welcomes input—and let's make this as enjoyable as we can." Team leaders can establish a positive tone immediately by greeting everyone by name and continuously inviting team members into conversation.

Ensure Psychological Safety

A critical component of setting the appropriate tone is ensuring team members' psychological safety. Within psychologically safe environments, everyone is comfortable speaking up, every individual and what they have to say is treated with respect at all times, and disrespectful actions are not tolerated.

Psychological safety is essential for teams,[8] as people act tentatively and defensively when they don't feel safe, thereby inhibiting their willingness to participate and speak up. When team members believe that they or their suggestions are being criticized, a very unhealthy dynamic occurs, eroding team cohesion.

Nothing can erode psychological safety faster than a disrespectful colleague. Such disrespectful behavior can lead to a decrease in contributions from other colleagues, a decrease in task performance from other colleagues, and an increase in the general negative mood and anger of the room. In short, there is no place for unprofessional disruptive behavior in a team—it's dangerous.[9]

As previously mentioned, to ensure psychological safety, leaders must be very explicit that overt disrespect is not acceptable and will not be tolerated. To do this, organizations must codify respect into the credentialing process and deal with violations to that code consistently and swiftly. Is leadership willing to codify this in the credentialing process and hold individuals equally accountable regardless of their standing and how much business they bring in? If so, a high-performance, safe culture can be achieved; if not, the chances of having a serious, avoidable, and potentially indefensible event rises dramatically.

Consider this example. An organization had been working with its entire surgical staff on teamwork and communication skills. The hospital had instituted multiple initiatives to improve communication, and organization leadership was proud of their accomplishments and believed that the organization supported teamwork and communication.

One day during a particularly stressful procedure, a surgeon lost his temper with the circulating nurse. According to the surgeon, the nurse was not moving fast enough and was "slowing him down" by asking him to clarify a situation. His tone turned hostile. The nurse continued to ask for clarification, and the surgeon picked up the closest thing to him—a bloody sponge—and flung it at her, yelling for her to just stop talking for one minute so he could think. The tone in the room got very quiet, and the surgeon completed the procedure shortly after. After the procedure was finished, the nurse and her colleagues reported the event to their supervisors and the organization's patient safety officer. Although the physician received a warning, he was never asked to apologize to the nurse, and the consequences of his actions were not immediately seen. Rumors of this event spread through the entire organization, and in a manner of weeks, all the teamwork and communication efforts the hospital leadership had so painstakingly encouraged were for naught. Leaders had inadvertently sent the message that teamwork and communication were important for some but not for others, and when push came to shove, if you were smart, talented, and brought business to the hospital, you could behave in any way you wanted. Nursing staff members learned once again that it was better to keep your mouth shut than to express an opinion, and the operating room returned to its previous levels of ineffective communication and teamwork.

If an organization believes in creating a safe work environment in which all employees are treated with respect at all times, then it needs to be very clear that management will consistently model those values, send the message that anything less is not acceptable, and actively intervene in a timely manner to deal with disrespectful behavior. Let's look at a different example:

A neurosurgeon showed up for a case one day in a bad mood, refused to engage in the perioperative briefing for the case, and was rude to the nurses. At the end of the procedure, when he left the operating room, the CEO, the chief medical officer, and the patient safety physician were all waiting for him. The conversation was very short and to the point, "Fred, I don't know what's wrong with you today, but you know better than this—get your butt back in that room and apologize to the nurses." The fact that leadership rapidly intervened, the desired behaviors were strongly reinforced, and an apology was delivered to the nurses within minutes sent a very powerful message within the organization.

Use Structured Communication Techniques

Communication between individuals is often informal, disorganized, and variable. In situations where specific and complex information must be communicated and responded to in a timely manner, and the consequences of omitting critical information can be dire, it is essential to add structure to the exchange. Such structure can ensure that the right information is shared at the right time with the right people. Following are some specific structured communication techniques that all patient care teams should use:

Briefings

Briefings are a critical element in team effectiveness and determine whether people work together as a cohesive team or as a group of individuals with different ideas and goals sharing the same space. They quickly help set the tone for team interaction, ensure that people providing clinical care have a shared mental model of what's going to happen during a process, identify any risk points, plan for contingencies, and avoid surprises. When done effectively, briefings can establish predictability, reduce interruptions, prevent delays, and build social relationships and capital for future interactions.[10]

When structuring a briefing, it is important to keep in mind certain key elements, including the following (*see* Sidebar 6-1 on page 53 for a checklist for briefings):

• Be concise. For briefings to add value, they have to be seen as providing a positive return for the time spent. Meaningful information should be communicated quickly, enhancing operational efficiency, not hindering it.

• Involve others. Having a two-way conversation during a briefing is essential. Engaging others and explicitly asking for their input and suggestions brings more expertise to the issue at hand. A two-way conversation also offers an opportunity to assess people's comfort level and prior experience relative to a clinical task. Having team members participate enhances team formation and clarifies that everyone has a responsibility to insure safe care and speak up if they perceive something to be unsafe.

• Use first names. Familiarity is a key factor in the willingness of people to speak up when they perceive a problem. If you are in an environment in which people don't know each other, write names on a whiteboard for reference.

• Make eye contact and face the person. As the Buddhists would say—be in the moment. Acknowledging others and paying attention to what they say sends a positive message, thus reinforcing that their contributions have value and importance. It is important to note that eye contact should be exercised when working with individuals who are culturally comfortable with it. Some cultures view direct eye contact as a threat and thus it should be avoided in situations where a team member is uncomfortable.[4]

While briefings can and should be done in almost any situation, there are some environments in which briefings are particularly important, including the following:

• **In procedural areas.** In this environment, briefing

Sidebar 6-1. Checklist for a Concise Briefing

Following is a checklist that team leaders can use to help ensure that a briefing is thorough yet concise[4]:

✔ I got the other person's attention.

✔ I made eye contact and faced the person.

✔ I introduced myself and used people's names—familiarity is key.

✔ I shared the plan and asked for information they would know.

✔ I explicitly asked for input—both expertise and concerns.

✔ We talked about next steps.

✔ I encouraged ongoing monitoring and cross-checking.

---

prior to each procedure should be done. As previously mentioned, such briefing should include a discussion of the plan, contingencies to the plan, possible risk points, and so forth. As part of its Universal Protocol for Preventing Wrong Site, Wrong Procedure, Wrong Person Surgery™, The Joint Commission requires surgical teams to conduct a specific type of preprocedure briefing—typically called a time-out—in which the correct site, patient, and procedure are verified. This briefing is also an opportunity to address other issues such as antibiotic administration, medications, allergies, access to critical equipment, anticipated problems, and other salient issues. The World Health Organization (WHO) has released a Surgical Safety Checklist for preprocedure briefings (*see* Chapter 13, page 118, for more details).

The WHO Surgical Safety Checklist and the High-5 Correct Site Surgery Standard Operating Protocol (due in 2009; please check the WHO Collaborating Centre for Patient Safety Solutions Web site at http://www.ccforpatientsafety.org/ for information and updates) both seek to improve the safety of surgical procedures. As a result, they have many features in common. However, although they are not identical, they are compatible with each other. The High-5 protocol focuses specifically on reducing the risk of wrong-patient, wrong-procedure, wrong-site surgery in certain types of surgical cases and requires participating hospitals to adhere to the protocol as written, to measure their performance and share their results. In contrast, the WHO Surgical Safety Checklist addresses a much broader array of surgical risks, is available to any organization wishing to use it, and is presented as a model tool that may be modified at the user's discretion to

fit local practice. Where the two documents overlap—certain preoperative checks, site marking, and the "time-out" before surgery—the expectations are consistent. Where they differ is in the range of perioperative activities included in each. The High-5 protocol has a more fully developed preoperative verification process that begins when the surgical procedure is first scheduled and continues throughout the preoperative process, while the WHO checklist is initiated preoperatively on the day of surgery. On the other hand, the WHO checklist includes a postoperative "sign out" process that is not part of the High-5 protocol. All of these components have value and, indeed, should be implemented by all organizations providing surgical services.

In addition to the preprocedure briefing, team members should consider spending a few minutes at the beginning of the day to look across the schedule, anticipate equipment and supply needs, and plan for contingencies. This is not only time well spent, but it allows each preprocedural briefing to be shorter, can prevent delays in starting procedures, and can minimize interruptions during procedures. There are times when procedures are significantly delayed because the team doesn't have all the tools, equipment, and supplies it needs for the operation. Sometimes a specific tool is not even in the hospital, and the procedure is held up while the tool is brought on site. This can be a risk to patient safety and is completely preventable. By conducting a briefing before the start of a schedule, team members can identify what special equipment and supplies are needed, and that equipment and those supplies can be brought in before the procedure begins. (*See* Sidebar 6-2 on page 54.) Such planning can also minimize the need for the circulating nurse to leave the OR to retrieve necessary equipment and supplies during a procedure. When a circulating nurse leaves the OR, it is not only a distraction to the procedure but it may present an infection control risk as well.[11]

• **In the Intensive Care Unit (ICU).** Given the intensity and frequently changing nature of the patient needs in the ICU, it is important that teams come together at the beginning of the day and periodically throughout the day to talk about patients, plans of care, possible risk points, and issues to watch. This can help all team members get on the same page and see the big picture of what patients need what care in what time frame. The use of multidisciplinary rounds and setting daily goals for each patient should be a fundamental goal in the ICU.[12]

• **In ambulatory care.** With the high volume and short intervals involved with this type of care, it is constructive to take a few minutes in the morning to brief the day's activities. Within such a briefing, some things to discuss could include here's who's coming in, here's who we're concerned about, and here's the information we need. Team members should identify which patients should be simple, and who is probably going to be complicated. In addition to the morning briefing, the team should briefly reconnect at points throughout the day to address questions such as How are we doing on time? Who's new? What's different? This helps keep everyone in "the same movie," a set of shared context and expectations. Such a briefing is much more effective than the typical one-on-one hallway conversations that can occur within the ambulatory care setting.

• **On the spot/as the situation changes.** If something significantly changes in the course of patient care, team leaders should take a few moments to make sure everyone is working off a common mental model.

• **Handoffs.** These occur when patient care is transferred from one team member to another. These are inherently dangerous times, as critical information can be lost, forgotten, or misinterpreted during handoffs. A high percentage of errors occur at transitions of care. Handoffs may take place in a variety of situations. They may involve one service taking over for another in the emergency department, such as gynecology for general surgery in a patient with pelvic pain; or a physical handoff, such as moving from the postoperative recovery room to the ICU. No matter what the type of handoff, it is important that pertinent information is effectively communicated and does not get lost in the shuffle. To ensure effective handoff communications, your organization may want to use structured language (*see* pages 56–58). In addition, to make sure all the appropriate information is communicated every time, you may want to use tools such as checklists. Within its National Patient Safety Goals, The Joint Commission requires organizations to have a structured process for patient handoffs to ensure effective communication.

Debriefings

While briefings typically occur before a process, procedure, schedule of procedures, and so forth, a debriefing is a concise exchange that occurs after such events have been completed to identify what happened, what was learned, and what can be done better next time.[13] It is a valuable

Sidebar 6-2. Gaining Physician Support for Briefings

As previously mentioned, fostering collaboration through briefings is not innate to many physicians. In some cases, it goes against the very fiber of their being. However, physicians' participation in and leadership of briefings is critical—particularly in the operating room. To gain physician support, organizations may want to pitch the concept of briefings in terms that the physician values.

1. If you conduct briefings, your day will run smoother. You will have the equipment you need, when you need it, and everyone will be working together to achieve common goals.

2. If you conduct briefings, patients will be safer, and so will you. Because of the structured communication involved in briefings and the effective communication that results from briefings, patient harm is less likely, continuous learning can be achieved, and malpractice risk is reduced.

opportunity rarely used in medicine to determine how participants in a team are feeling about the process and identify opportunities for improvement as well as further education and learning. Debriefing is also an effective venue for problem solving and generating new solutions—often with ideas brought from other clinical domains by the experts on the team. It is a very good way to positively engage the collective wisdom of a care team.

The effectiveness of a debriefing is dependent on the effectiveness of the briefing. If you weren't clear at the front end, you won't be able to effectively wrap up information. The debriefing conversation should be focused on the common goal and have a positive tone. In facilitating a debriefing, team leaders should be as specific as possible. It's nice to say "nice job," but not much is learned. The more specific and detailed, the more value will be gained. Appropriate questions to ask during debriefing include:

• What did we do well? Focus on both individual and team tasks.

• What did we learn?

• What would we do differently next time?

• Were there system issues like equipment problems or incomplete information that made our job more difficult? Who's going to own the system problems so they will get fixed and not be a recurrent pebble in our shoe next time?

During debriefing it is important to engage the most junior team members first. If you engage the 20-year veteran nurse first, and she says she did not see any issues, the nurse fresh out of nursing school may be hesitant to bring up an issue. However, if you ask the recent graduate first, you not only encourage him or her to speak freely and identify potential issues but also help him or her learn and grow professionally.

As a result of debriefing, teams should document items that did not go well and make suggestions for improvement. As discussed in Chapter 5, such documentation should be tied to the spontaneous reporting system or "glitch book" in which team members write down a problem that needs fixing. By documenting problems, teams can take a step toward fixing them and preventing issues down the line.

Debriefings can not only identify problems to fix, but they can speed up team learning. Such learning can occur regardless of the experience of the team leader. For example, a recent study by Bohmer et al. showed that when learning a new cardiac surgery procedure, the team that had the shortest learning curve and greatest outcomes was led by a junior cardiac surgeon. This was due in part because this surgeon conducted a debriefing after every operation and created an environment of organizational learning within his team.[6]

SBAR Model

An acronym for Situation, Background, Assessment, Recommendation, this structured communication technique is used to standardize communication between two or more people.[14] It helps set the expectation within a conversation that specific, relevant, and critical informational elements are going to be communicated every time a patient is discussed. The SBAR model is particularly helpful in situations where a nurse-physician encounter must occur. It helps get both parties on the same page, as the physicians want to focus on the problem and the solution, and the nurses know they will be expected to relate specific aspects of the problem. SBAR sets the expectation that critical thinking associated with defining the patient's problem and formulating a solution occur before the physician is contacted. Thus both parties know that the conversation will include the assessment and recommendation for care that is relevant to the patient's current status.

Following is a description of steps involved in SBAR:

• *Situation.* This is the part of the mechanism in which the two parties communicating establish the topic of which they are going to speak.

• *Background.* This is any information needed to make an informed decision for the patient, including the following:

—The admitting diagnosis and date of admission

—List of current medications, allergies, intravenous fluids, and labs

—Most recent vital signs

—Lab results, with the date and time the test was performed, and results of previous tests for comparison

—Other clinical information

—Code status

• *Assessment.* The individual initiating the SBAR should state an assessment of the situation and the patient's status.

• *Recommendation.* The individual initiating the SBAR should offer a recommendation of what to do next and when it should happen.

The following dialogue illustrates how a respiratory therapist can use the SBAR model to communicate with a physician regarding a patient's situation:

• *Situation.* "I'm calling about Ms. Jones, who is short of breath."

• *Background.* "She's a patient with chronic lung disease; she's been sliding downhill; and she's now acutely worse."

• *Assessment.* "She has decreased breath sounds on the right side. I think she's probably collapsed a lung."

• *Recommendation.* "I think she needs a chest tube. I need you to come see her now. When will you be here?"

In this example, the respiratory therapist effectively communicates using the SBAR model. The communication is concise, clear, and resulted in timely action.

Assertive Language

Because medicine has an inherent hierarchal structure and power distances between individuals, it is critically important that health care workers politely assert themselves in the name of safety. Effective assertion is pleasant and persistent; it is not a license to be aggressive, hostile, or confrontational. This type of communication is also timely, clear, and offers solutions to presenting problems.

As previously mentioned, numerous high-profile accidents in medicine and elsewhere have demonstrated that in many cases team members knew that "something didn't seem right," but their ability to speak up and clearly communicate was inhibited. Often, the information was relayed in an oblique and indirect manner. The whole concept of "hint and hope"—"I said something, they must have heard it, and everything will be OK"— is all too common.

When assertion is ineffective, a look back usually reveals the following:

- Concern was expressed.
- The problem was stated in an oblique and indirect way.
- A proposed action didn't happen.
- A decision was not reached.

Organizations can help ensure appropriate assertion in team communication by training staff in assertion techniques. A formal checklist can be used to help staff learn a positive way to assert their opinions. Following is an example of such a checklist:

- Get the person's attention.
- Make eye contact, face the person.
- Use the person's name.
- Express concern.
- State the problem clearly and concisely.
- Propose action.
- Make sure the problem and proposed action are understood by all parties.
- Reassert as necessary.
- Reach decision.
- Make sure decision is understood by all parties—do a readback.
- Escalate if necessary.

By following this checklist, staff members can ensure that their point is made. An individual may not always get the decision he or she wants, but at least everyone will be having the same conversation. It may be helpful to practice the use of such a checklist during role playing exercises.

Critical Language

During a stressful situation, such as within a surgical procedure or intense patient care episode, not everyone will immediately think of the most appropriate way to get people's attention and communicate information effectively—particularly if the person needing to get people's attention is hesitant to speak up due to hierarchy issues, his or her cultural background, or lack of psychological safety.

Often providers, such as physicians, may not be aware of a situation, and using nondirect language may not be strong enough to signal a problem. For this reason, it can be helpful to empower professionals with critical language that when spoken indicates to other team members that work should cease and all attention be focused on the speaker.

Such language may include a phrase like "I need a little clarity," a wonderful, neutral term that came from Allina Hospitals. A request for "clarity" can be used in the presence of a patient and his or her family, and all caregivers know that what is really being said is "let's just take a minute and make sure we are doing the right thing." Teams that respond to critical language know there is a concern that needs to be immediately addressed, and all work should cease until that situation is resolved.

Critical language should be neutral, help focus on doing the right thing, and foster a situation in which no one believes that their competence or expertise is being questioned.

Consider this example. A surgeon is preparing to perform knee surgery on an elderly patient. Although he has verified the medical record, he is distracted and tired—this is his fourth knee surgery of the day, and there have been other issues with this patient that have diverted his attention. As he prepares to operate on the knee, a nurse in the room notices the surgeon's scalpel is hovering over the incorrect knee. This is the hospital's most prominent orthopedic surgeon, and the nurse is concerned about bringing up an issue. The nurse clears her throat and says, "Excuse me, doctor, but I need some clarity about the knee on which you are going to operate." The physician, along with everyone else in the room, knows that this is a cue to stop, brief about the situation, and ensure that everyone is comfortable. As he stops, the physician realizes his error and moves to the correct knee. The team performs a quick verification[15] of the correct patient, site, and side and proceeds with the operation.

Common Language

In some settings, using a common language, which is agreed upon by all providers in that setting, to describe critical issues or observations may be helpful to ensure consistency yet comprehensiveness in communication. For example, within the obstetrics setting, communication about fetal heart tracing can often be confusing and misleading. Different providers have different ways of expressing concern. When a fetal tracing indicates a problem, providers must move quickly and efficiently. Wasting time deciphering what someone means is not a luxury that the situation affords. To help clarify communication among providers about fetal heart tracings, The National Institute of Child Health and Human Development has defined an agreed common language in obstetrics that describes such tracings. By committing to using this language, organizations can ensure consistent communication about a critical issue across all types of providers and within many different types of situations. More about fetal heart tracing language can be found in Chapter 13.

Closed Communication Loops

A closed communication loop helps improve the reliability of communication by having the person receiving the communication restate what the sender has said to confirm understanding. One specific type of closed loop communication is repeat back. The tool involves four distinct actions:

1. The "sender" concisely states information to the "receiver."

2. The receiver then repeats back what he or she heard.

3. The sender then acknowledges the repeat back was correct or makes a correction.

4. The process continues until a shared understanding is verified. Within this model, responding to a message with an "okay" or an "uh-huh" is not sufficient to close the communication loop. The message must be explicitly restated and acknowledged.

Organizations requiring this type of closed-loop communication during times in which communication must be reliable and effective can help smooth the communication process and ensure no critical information is lost. Closed-loop communication can be particularly helpful in situations such as during surgery to confirm sponge count, during high-risk patient handoffs to ensure comprehensive information exchange, and during medication ordering to ensure that the right medication, right dose, and right route are communicated. The Joint Commission addresses this issue by requiring organizations to use a read-back closed communication process when confirming verbal or telephone orders. (*See* Sidebar 6-3, above.)

Active Listening

A critical component of communication is listening. If providers do not listen to one another, then they can't effectively exchange information. Conversation is a two-way exercise involving both speaking and listening. Active listening is a concept in which a provider approaches the act of listening in the following way:

• Maintains a comfortable level of eye contact

• Monitors body language—both his or her own and the speaker's—to ensure that the correct messages are being sent

---

Sidebar 6-3. National Patient Safety Goal 2

Through National Patient Safety Goal (NPSG) 2, The Joint Commission requires organizations to institute a verbal read-back process for verbal or telephone orders or for telephone reporting of critical test results. Within this process, the individual giving the order must verify the complete order or test result by having the person receiving the information record and "read back" the complete order or test result.

To further prevent errors associated with verbal and written orders, NPSG 2 requires organizations to create a standardized list of abbreviations, acronyms, symbols, and dose designations that are not to be used throughout the organization, including within verbal or written orders.

---

and received

• Listens completely without framing a response while the individual is still speaking

• Repeats back information to confirm understanding

Callouts

Typically used in procedural settings, callouts involve clearly spoken phrases that indicate a phase of a process. This technique is often used in the OR at two points—the start of a procedure and the closing. Surgical teams may also use the callout technique at other times, such as to say the sponge count is correct or the patient is coming off bypass. Some further examples of callouts include the following:

• "We're closing."

• "I'm going to need X-ray in about 20 minutes."

• "We'll be done in 30 minutes."

• "We're bleeding more than I like—we may need to open. We'll decide within five minutes."

When using the callout technique, participants should speak clearly and loudly so all team members can hear.

Create Situational Awareness

Situational awareness (SA) is defined as a shared understanding of "what's going on," "what is likely to happen next," and "what to do if what is supposed to happen doesn't."[4] SA requires that team members have a common mental model of what is really expected. By maintaining situational awareness, the care team creates a common understanding of what they are trying to accomplish; monitors and reports progress or potential problems; and avoids "tunnel vision"—becoming fixated on a particular task rather than the "larger picture"—to ensure that progress conforms to the shared model.

Within a complicated and hectic health care process, such as a surgical procedure or an ICU intervention, SA is easily lost, and the risk of accidents and problems goes up dramatically. Certain "red flags" can indicate the loss or potential loss of SA and the presence of any of the following red flags[4] should alert team members that risk is increasing and should be discussed.

- *Things don't feel right.* This is probably the most important indicator of a problem. Individuals pattern-match against previous experience. If intuition is telling an individual there is a problem, then the chances are quite good that the team is getting in trouble. If the hair on the back of his or her neck is standing up, or he or she is getting a bad feeling about what's going on, then the individual should verbalize any concerns to other team members so the problem can be addressed.

- *Ambiguity.* If it is becoming less clear what the plan is, then the team needs to talk to make sure they are on the same page. It's hard to monitor the plan if team members are not sure what is supposed to be happening.

- *Reduced/poor communication.* Faced with a problem, effective teams and leaders consciously enhance and increase communication. Raising concerns, gathering input, agreeing on how to approach problems, and having team members verify results should increase during problematic situations

- *Confusion*

- *Trying something new under pressure.* This reflects the sense that the practitioner(s) does not have a workable approach to the problem at hand. It's far more successful to stay with the tried and true approach, used many times before, than to launch into novel approaches under duress. This is not to say being creative and innovative is not a positive attribute, however when a team is behind the curve, they should do what they do best.

- *Deviating from established norms.* Norms have been established because they often reflect safe approaches to care. Unless there is a clear and compelling benefit discussed and clarified by the team, this can be an indicator of a problem.

- *Verbal violence.* This is a proxy for frustration. Effective communication becomes difficult when someone is being verbally unpleasant. It also affects people's comfort level in speaking up or questioning the current approach.

- *Fixation.* When people become task fixated, they lose the ability to see the context of the situation. An example of this would be the physician, who is so fixated on getting the difficult central line in that he fails to notice the patient is becoming hypoxic or unstable.

- *Boredom.* It takes conscious work to maintain vigilance and attention. When bored, it is easy for one's mind to wander from the task at hand. Being on autopilot is a good way to miss critical information.

- *Task saturation.* Being busy and feeling overwhelmed indicates a need to ask for help and communicate with other team members. Being behind the curve and working hard to keep up narrows an individual's ability to process important information.

- *Being rushed/behind schedule.* In today's busy world of medical practice, everyone feels rushed or behind at some point. The danger with this situation is that it is human nature to cut corners when behind, and something important may be missed. Given that being rushed is something that is encountered frequently, the safest answer is for individuals to check in with fellow team members to see that they are not missing something that could adversely affect patient care.

Building and maintaining SA is a collective process involving the entire team. Teams that take the following actions can establish and maintain SA:

- Communicate in a concise, specific, and timely manner.

- Use briefings and ongoing updates to ensure that every team member knows the game plan.

- Acknowledge and demonstrate common understanding using repeat-back procedures.

- Talk to one another as events unfold so the team can monitor and verify perspectives.

- Anticipate the next steps and discuss possible contingencies.

- Constructively assert opinions and perspectives.

- Verbalize red flags if they are present.

STRUCTURES THAT ENHANCE TEAMWORK AND COMMUNICATION

In addition to the previously mentioned strategies and skills, organizations can and should establish structures in which effective teamwork and communication can take place. Following is a discussion of two such structures.

Multidisciplinary Rounds

An effective way to incorporate all the previously mentioned structured communication techniques is to use multidisciplinary rounds. These are rounds in which every member of the care team is present and every patient is discussed. When possible, the patient and family are included on these rounds. Such rounds should take place at least twice a day at shift changes, and an abbreviated version should occur throughout the day to address new developments, changes, or problematic situations. Within these rounds, teams should discuss the plan of care for each patient. As previously mentioned, teams can use structured communication techniques, such as SBAR, briefings, and common language, to help facilitate and streamline rounding conversations. Teams may also consider using whiteboards to spur discussion of every patient.

While rounding can be effective in many different environments, it can be particularly useful in the obstetrics department and emergency department. Within these two departments, staff cannot control patient volume and thus can benefit from periodically coming together, discussing risks, anticipating problems, and communicating when workload is getting too much. When a staff member is feeling overwhelmed by his or her patient load, he or she should feel empowered to speak up during rounds, so work can be reallocated to ensure the safety of patients.

Red Rules

Red rules, as adopted by Sentara Norfolk General Hospital from the nuclear power industry, are non-negotiable rules that, except in rare, urgent situations, should always be followed.[16] For example, a red rule in construction is "always wear a hard hat on the job site." A red rule in transportation safety is "always have children wear seat belts when riding in a car." Red rules in surgery are "always conduct a time-out to verify the correct patient, procedure, and site before surgery" and "if there is any indication we are missing something, never leave the operating room without an X-ray." A red rule in obstetrics is "if the nurse or midwife asks a physician to come see a patient, the physician comes, 100% of the time."

Establishing red rules is important because it communicates to everyone involved in a process how important that process is and how the organization values the performance of that process. Establishing and enforcing red rules can help

ensure that the proper care is given 100% of the time and thus can improve patient safety.

To be effective, red rules must be agreed upon by everyone in the organization from the board of directors down to the frontline staff. They must be developed collaboratively and enforced consistently. There should be no ambiguity about the process and its necessity. Everyone who works at the hospital should know that performing this process is not a judgment call, but an absolute, nonnegotiable requirement. If an individual, such as a surgeon or physician, blows off a red rule, there should be immediate, observable consequences. There is no excuse for doing something that is consciously unsafe.

Within your organization's accountability system, providers should be held 100% accountable for violating a red rule and face disciplinary action, such as losing their license if such a rule is violated.

Your organization should have only one or two red rules per setting, so that it is clear that these rules are inviolate and must be followed 100% of the time. If every process involves a red rule, then the importance of the red rule is lessened, and compliance with the red rule will go down.

Another key aspect to the success of red rules is education. Everyone involved in the process must be educated in a variety of ways on what the red rule is, why it is important, and what the consequences will be if the rule is not followed.

TRAINING FOR EFFECTIVE TEAMWORK AND COMMUNICATION

Strong team performance with an emphasis on two-way communication, respect, idea sharing, and problem solving is essential to the safe and reliable delivery of care. Not only do health care teams not typically have this type of interaction, but many members of the team are unaware of how poor their communication and team behaviors are. For example, if you ask a physician if communication in care teams is effective, he or she will mostly likely say "yes." However, if you ask nurses the same question, you will get a different answer. In fact, 25%–40% of nurses surveyed using a cultural assessment tool say they would be hesitant to speak up if they saw a physician making a mistake.[17] Part of the reason for this is that physicians and nurses view teamwork differently. Nurses believe good teamwork exists when they are asked for their input and feedback. Physicians believe it exists when everyone does what they say.

Effective teamwork and communication skills are not necessarily something a person is born with. Yes, there are those truly gifted individuals who have almost a sixth sense about what to say when and how. However, for the rest of us, communication strategies and teamwork skills can and should be taught, practiced, and reinforced until they become second nature and a critical part of how we operate. Unfortunately, in medicine, teamwork and communication skills have not commonly been included in the curriculum of medical, nursing, pharmacy, or other health care schools. And so, the responsibility for such education falls on the health care organization.

The best way to train providers on teamwork and communication is to bring them together in multidisciplinary sessions; communicate the need for teamwork and communication; educate them on team behaviors, communication strategies, and structures for communication using scenarios they understand and can relate to; and have them practice using the behaviors and strategies. With this approach, two things happen. One is procedural learning—"I have done this, and I know how to do it well." This is extremely important in a culture that keeps score by knowing the answers and doing things well. People are far more likely to do something back at the bedside if they have practiced.

The second thing that happens is social agreement. When physicians, nurses, and technicians discuss a real case and how they would communicate about it and respond, they reach consensus about the appropriate communication pattern and practice together. This is very powerful in forming and enhancing relationships, the foundation of a safer culture.

As discussed in Chapter 2, before officially starting a training session, you may want to consider administering the safety culture assessment survey, realizing a high response rate is critical to success in assessing a culture, and a team training session has a committed, multidisciplinary audience that can ensure effective survey administration.

At the beginning of the training session, to help draw in providers, it is helpful to use a story to engage their participation and make the topic "real." Throughout the training you should focus on what their perceptions of teamwork are and how observations of their environment show a different story (see Chapter 7 for more information on observing teamwork and communication).

To be successful, these training sessions should have ALL members of the care team present, including physicians. Those organizations serious about enhancing teamwork and communication make it mandatory for everyone to attend. In organizations where physicians are employees, making teamwork training sessions mandatory is fairly straightforward. Those organizations with licensed independent practitioners may have more of a challenge, but creative approaches can help solicit physician participation. For example, one organization offered a stipend for every physician who practices in the hospital to attend team training. By doing this, they were then able to make attendance mandatory. Another hospital tied participation in teamwork training to the credentialing process and made it a requirement for physicians to attend. Although involving physicians in team training can be challenging, if you don't involve them, then all the teamwork training in the world will not enhance the dynamics of the care team and improve safety.

REFERENCES

1. Reinertsen J.L.: Zen and the art of physician autonomy maintenance. *Ann Int Med* 138:992–995, 2003.
2. Bosk C.L.: *Forgive and remember: Managing medical failure.* Chicago: University of Chicago Press, 1979.
3. Detert J.R., Edmondson A.C.: Everyday failures in organizational learning: Explaining the high threshold for speaking up at work. Harvard Business School Faculty Working Papers http://www.hbs.edu/research/pdf/06-024.pdf (accessed Nov.9, 2008).
4. Leonard M., Frankel A., Simmonds T.: *Achieving safe and reliable healthcare.* Chicago: Health Administration Press, 2004.
5. Joint Commision *Sentinel Event Alert* 40, Jul. 9, 2008. http://www.jointcommission.org/SentinelEvents/SentinelEventAlert/sea_40.htm (accessed Nov. 9, 2008).
6. Edmondson A.C., Bohmer R., Pisano G.P.: Speeding up team learning. *Harvard Business Review* Oct. 1, 2001.
7. Mazzocco K., Petitti D.B., Fong K.T., et al.: Surgical team behaviors and patient outcomes. *The American Journal of Surgery*, 2008, in press.
8. Edmondson A.C.: Managing the risk of learning: Psychological safety in work teams; West, M. (Ed) *International Handbook of Organizational Teamwork*, London: Blackwell, 2002.
9. Rosenstein A.H., Russell H., Lauve R.: Disruptive physician behavior contributes to nursing shortage. *Physician Executive* pp. 8–11, Nov.–Dec. 2002.
10. Makary M.A., et al.: Operating room briefings: Working on the same page. *Jt Comm J Qual Patient Saf* 32:351–355, Jun. 2006.
11. Reduced risk of prosthetic infections thanks to behavioral and technical measures taken in operating room. University Medical Center Groningen http://www.umcg.nl/azg/nl/english/nieuws/87062 (accessed Nov. 9, 2008).
12. Pronovost P.J, et al.: Implementing and validating a comprehensive unit-based safety program. *J Pat Safety* 1:33–40, 2005.
13. Makary M.A., et al.: Operating room debriefings. *J Qual Patient Saf* 32:407–410, Jul. 2006.
14. Haig K.M., Sutton S., Whittington J.: SBAR: A shared mental model for improving communication between clinicians. *Jt Comm J Qual Patient Saf* 32:167–175, Mar. 2006.
15. The Joint Commission: *Universal Protocol.* http://www.jointcommission.org/PatientSafety/UniversalProtocol (last accessed Sep. 3, 2008).
16. Yates G.R., et al.: Sentara Norfolk General Hospital: accelerating improvement by focusing on building a culture of safety. *Jt Comm J Qual Saf* 30:534–542, Oct. 2004.
17. Sexton J.B., Helmreich R.L., Neilands T.B., et al.: The Safety Attitudes Questionnaire: Psychometric properties, benchmarking data, and emerging research. *BMC Health Services Research* 6:44, Apr. 3, 2006.

Chapter Seven

USING DIRECT OBSERVATION AND FEEDBACK TO MONITOR TEAM PERFORMANCE

Allan Frankel and *Andrew Knight*

As discussed in Chapter 6, to improve performance of teams you must engage them in comprehensive and regular team training, which involves teaching communication strategies and skills, fostering interactions, engaging in role play, and practice, practice, practice.

A critical part of all change processes is measuring whether change has an effect, and so too, in efforts to improve teamwork the first question to ask, before asking about changes in clinical outcomes, is whether team training changes team behaviors. A common error is to focus immediately on whether the training will affect the work produced by the team. Ultimately that is the goal, although in reality teamwork should affect three aspects of the team—the work produced, the satisfaction derived from the team in performing that work, and the ability of the team to improve itself. Knowing first whether team training has had an effect and secondarily whether team work output has changed allows the two measurements to be related to each other and provides a reasonable degree of evidence that change in one influences the other.

One measure of team practice is whether the individuals who comprise the team perform the agreed-upon team behaviors and manifest the team norms of conduct. Careful observations of these team characteristics, quantified, can be held against team performance and adverse outcome rates (if measurable) and highlight performance by health care teams.

Historically this type of observation has tended to be performed in research settings using researchers who spend significant effort to learn the fundamentals of social psychology followed by extensive training in observation. Recently,

the authors of this book have moved from the perspective that observation is a research tool to a reframed perspective that observation should be feasible as a quality assessment tool. Frontline clinicians with some clinical expertise and careful training can observe team behaviors in real time and evaluate how teammates interact with one another, and how well they work together toward a common goal. Careful and focused training is making this a reality.

There are fundamental and definable components of assessing the effectiveness of interventions aimed at improving team skills. This type of data collection involves observing the essential characteristics of team behavior and leadership in a way that is accurate and reproducible.

People, in general, are highly sensitive social instruments, and each of us is naturally quite good at evaluating social environments, as evidenced by immediate awareness of the tension level or feeling of comfort that exists in a room when we walk into social situations. This applies to trained observers who can evaluate with reasonable reliability four characteristics of a clinical environment[1]:

- First, observers can note the physical characteristics that might increase risk, from something as obvious as wires or tubing on a floor presenting a tripping hazard to incomplete patient information in a chart.

- Second, observers can objectively and reproducibly observe specific defined behaviors, which will be discussed below.

- Third, observers can reproducibly characterize tension levels and whether they are appropriate for the situation.

- Fourth, observers may characterize leaders and their

ability to support team function.

As discussed in Chapter 2, the evaluation of culture, sometimes called climate, is perceived as an increasingly important component of improving the safety and reliability of health care organizations. The recent Joint Commission requirement that all hospitals perform safety culture surveys is evidence of this trend. Culture surveys can realistically be performed about every year and give a snapshot of attitudes, which combined produce the organization's culture.

Observation is another measurement of culture, and as both attitudinal survey measures and behavioral observation measures become better understood and refined, they will give overlapping images of the environment of care in which providers function.

In clinical settings from intensive care units (ICUs) to operating rooms (ORs) where teams do physical interventions and there is enough person-to-person interaction to make for a rich observation climate, it is feasible to link direct observation of tension levels and leadership to your organization's safety culture survey. This survey is based on providers self-report of a safety culture and is a snapshot of a brief time period of attitude.

Observation is based on a more objective perspective of culture, and multiple small observations, done serially over time, may offer a dynamic view of attitude. Senior leadership should look closely at these two types of data to get a picture of the safety and teamwork culture of different units within the organization.

The evidence for linking provider attitude and behaviors to real clinical outcomes is becoming increasingly persuasive, as evidenced by the Keystone project in Michigan where the most successful ICUs that achieved the lowest bloodstream infections secondary to central line placement were also the ICUs with the highest scores in teamwork.[2] In Southern California in the Kaiser hospitals,[3] teamwork behaviors have been recently linked to postoperative complications. These studies and others are generating a solid body of evidence to support the logic of monitoring and measuring attitude and behaviors and applying teamwork programs to improve them.[4]

HOW TO USE DIRECT OBSERVATION

Although nonmedical industries employ observation to monitor and improve team processes and communication,

the "gold standard" method for doing so in health care has yet to fully emerge but is well on its way.[5,6] To effectively observe team performance, you must have a systematic process in which trained observers measure performance using standardized definitions. When incorporating standards into your organization, consider the following points:

• How many observations should you do? How frequently? This will depend on the number of teams you are observing and the amount of data you want to collect. Formal observations of interventional areas require ongoing observation. One way to do this is to use sampling methods, such as a minimum of 5 observations per month—ideally 10–15. These 30-minute observations in areas such as the ORs, obstetric C-section suites, interventional radiology suites, and gastroeneterology suites. Another option would be concentrating observations over a two-month period and then repeating the observations some months later. However, the "right" number of observations done in this way has yet to be ascertained from current research.

• When should you observe? It is helpful to assess team performance both before and after team training. Observation efforts before team training can highlight differences between team members' perception of their behavior and reality. It can reveal areas of risk and opportunities for improvement. By sharing these differences with team members during team training programs, you can clearly illustrate the current picture and where the team needs to improve. This can encourage buy-in and participation in team training as well as awareness of the work that needs to be done.

Assessing team performance after team training helps measure the effect of training on the behaviors and efforts of the team. Are there differences in performance? Observing after team training can also help identify where posttraining efforts should focus. For example, teams may be doing reasonable briefings and time-outs but few end-of-process debriefings, in which case this important team behavior can be made a topic for further discussion by the unit.

• What should you observe? As mentioned above, observers are able to characterize environmental threats; specific team behaviors, such as briefings, read-backs, callouts, timeouts, Situation, Background, Assessment, Recommendation (SBAR), and so forth; specific team relationships and attitudes, such as respect and situational awareness; and leadership characteristics, such as motivating the team, seeking input, and resolving conflict. (*See* Sidebar 7-1 on page 68 for a more complete list.) Organizations can observe any or all of these; however, if you consider your observers to be like laboratory instruments, they understandably have capacity limits, and if used inappropriately will generate poor data. The key in observation is understanding the skills and limitations of your instruments, the observers, and designing observation methods to enhance inter-rater reliability while at the same time generating data that will be useful to the observed units and frontline providers.

• How elegantly you can define and describe what observers should look at makes an impact on how accurate their observations are. For example, good teams manifest situational awareness—knowing one's own actions relative to the whole, and, concurrently, being aware of the actions of others. Asking observers to evaluate situational awareness is tricky because, while there are some actions that might clue in the observer, situational awareness is a mind-set, and not necessarily observable. Make sure items are clearly defined to prevent confusion and problems with consistency. A proxy for situational awareness is offering help. If situational awareness and offering help are both on an observation sheet, it's unlikely that observers will be able to differentiate the one from the other.

• How should you observe? There are two primary ways of observing:

1. The checklist method. With this method, observers stand in the unit or patient care area and note the performance of team behaviors, such as read-backs, debriefings, callouts, and so forth. They look for whether the behavior occurs at the required or expected time (per observer evaluation), and they give each behavior a grade depending on how well the behavior was performed. When finished, observers can count the frequency of a behavior and assign a grade to the behavior by taking an average of the individual scores.

2. The gestalt method. This is akin to watching a sports team play a game and then assessing at the end how well the team played overall and performed the various functions that make up the sport. With this method, observers familiarize themselves with the behavioral metrics just prior to entering the clinical setting and then enter a unit for about 20 minutes and watch the provision of care. When they are finished watching, they leave and, looking at the list of metrics, identify what behaviors they saw. They grade those

behaviors in overview, summing mentally all the individual episodes into one and using a predetermined Likert scale. Interestingly enough, a trained observer can do just as good a job at scoring using the gestalt method as the checklist method.

• Who is going to conduct the observations? The simplest answer to this question is either domain experts or others. Domain experts—those individuals who work in the environment every day—will be more sensitive to the nuances of teamwork and communication behaviors but will be less objective. This is their department and their coworkers, and their perceptions of people are going to have inherent bias. On the good side, they will pick up subtle cues that a nondepartment member will miss, and they will understand clinical context, which is key to understanding complex relationships. However, they will also be accustomed to the status quo and desensitized to possibly glaring deficits. Consequently, you may opt, instead, to bring observers in from outside to do the observations. Although outside observers are more objective, they will be less sensitive, missing some of the issues and interactions that are more subtle.

To overcome the liabilities of both domain experts and others, you may choose to use both types of observers, which can help ensure that the observation is accurate, but may influence the rating reliability. Our experience suggests that the inter-rater reliability (*see* page 64). degradation is not that significant. What also tends to happen is that when the two types of observers are trained together, they tend to benefit from understanding each other's point of view. Often the greatest discrepancies between observers when they initially train together are the different perspectives on and awareness of patient involvement, clinician-patient interactions, and the teamwork process. Whether domain experts or others, some observers are very aware of how patients are engaged in the team dynamics, while others overlook the interactions with patients—until the topic is broached in training.

• How are you going to score the observations? Defining a consistent scoring system is critical to ensure observers rate performance reliably. Be realistic. Observers are not so sensitive that they will reliably give the same scores across a 10-point scale of excellence to poor team behaviors, and in truth, a 10-point scale is unnecessary to direct efforts to improve teamwork. Observers appear to do well when asked to characterize behaviors on a 4- or 5-point scale of unacceptable, poor, adequate, good, and excellent. Remember the purpose of observations—to identify those behaviors amenable to improvement, and to highlight those done well. A 4-point scale is adequate for this task.

• How are you going to train observers? Effective, comprehensive, and consistent training is key to achieving success with this data collection method. Observers must be trained in groups so that they can learn from each other.

One option for training involves using standardized videos of different scenarios, which are shown to groups who then score them, debrief, and compare their scores. Significant score differences are discussed so that varying points of view are highlighted. The videos are played over again, sometimes multiple times, in order to help the group develop standardized ways of looking at behaviors. In the process, individual observers become sensitized to their biases and instructed to keep these in mind when scoring. For example, some observers set unrealistic expectations for themselves and project those expectations onto those they observe. When their scores are lower than the rest of the training group, they are forced to reflect on their bias and adjust.

Occasionally, some individuals are attuned to the social environment so differently that they are unable to come in line with the observer group, and it's reasonable to not use these individuals as observers. Some of us do see things differently! Showing all observers a standardized set of videos enables everyone to receive the same training on what to observe, how to observe, and how to score what is observed. Although organizations may need to devote several days to this training to ensure that trainers are trained thoroughly and appropriately, we have had success in training groups of domain experts and nonclinicians in about half a day—if the training is well orchestrated and efficient.

• How are you going to ensure inter-rater reliability? In the context of observation, inter-rater reliability is the level of agreement between two observers. When inter-rater reliability is good, two observers will grade team performance in a similar way. When it is not good, observers will vary in their grading, skewing the results and degrading measurement accuracy. It is important to both establish and maintain inter-rater reliability. Good training is key to establishing such reliability.

To maintain reliability, observers must perform paired observations during which they will need to follow a stricter set of rules than in normal observations. A simple example explains why. If two observers enter an OR and move to separate parts of the room, or even stand side by side but see different parts of the room, then they are likely to observe different sets of interactions. One might see the anesthesiologist in discussion with a nurse, while the other may see the surgeon and scrub technician speaking to each other. If the two observers compare notes afterward they will have seen different parts of the procedure, and their results will be different. Observers testing inter-rater reliability should agree to focus on similar team actions and then discuss only those activities.

• How are you going to analyze data collected during observation? Turning completed observation sheets into simply understandable reports is key. The two characteristics that can be documented for each observed metric are frequency and quality. While quality is always important, the utility of frequency varies. For example, when observing the beginning of a procedure, it is probably reasonable to expect that a briefing will be observed and scored. If no briefing occurs, that is significant. If a briefing is seen, identifying its quality is the next measurement.

On the other hand, most units would be deeply troubled to see a conflict resolution score on every observation sheet, regardless of the quality, as that would imply that conflict was an endemic characteristic of the unit. Equally troublesome, however, is periodic scoring of unresolved conflict, indicating that while the team generally gets along well, when it doesn't, lacking are the skills to address the issues.

• How are you going to share data with patient care teams and leaders? Sharing information is a key component to getting buy-in for improvement efforts and for giving feedback when improvement efforts are under way. By graphically displaying the different spectrum of scores, you can visually communicate the effectiveness of team performance and areas of improvement. This can provide motivation for improvement and reinforce desired behaviors.

METHODS OF DIRECT OBSERVATION

The following sections discuss two current models for direct observation.

The TICOT Model for Direct Observation

Building on research models from crisis resource management and applying insights from the social and cognitive psychology literature, the Teamwork in Context Observation Tool (TICOT) model evaluates threats, team behaviors, team relationships, and leadership characteristics in interventional teams. The one-page metric attempts to triangulate three conflicting tensions: the ability of human beings to observe and characterize social events; the limits of the human mind to track multiple variables at one time; and the desire to keep observation as a simple tool for quality evaluations, affordable in the health care climate.

As mentioned above, humans are thoroughly social beings with sensitized antennae for how individuals interact with each other. However, like all quality instruments, humans must be focused in the right direction and periodically "recalibrated." Within the TICOT Model, the questions asked of the observers are similar, and in some cases identical, to the questions on the Safety Attitudes Questionnaire discussed in Chapter 2. This was done to facilitate linking of the attitudinal survey scores with observed team relationships.

Within the TICOT model, there are 21 observable metrics, with testing to date suggesting there is little overlap between the definitions, a key requirement to maintain inter-rater reliability. However, fine-tuning is necessary during observation training—for example, agreeing upon the difference between a briefing and sharing information. (A briefing is a more formal coming together of some or all of the group to ensure that the game plan is understood, while sharing information is less formal and may consist of only pieces of the whole game plan).

Finally, the TICOT is designed to be completed after about a 20–40 minute observation period.

The TICOT questions are divided into four categories:

- Operational context
- Team climate and process
- Behaviors
- Leadership

Operational context evaluates the threats that, when evident, increase risk or decrease reliability of care. Observers are asked to rate the following statements[3]:

1. The physical environment supported safe care.

2. Equipment and materials were available and worked well.

3. Expertise not within the team was effectively accessed when needed.

4. All the necessary information for diagnostic and therapeutic decisions—history, labs, tests— was available when needed.

5. Interruptions and distractions were rare.

6. Staffing was sufficient to handle the workload.[3]

Team climate and process evaluates team member relationships using the following statements:

1. Team members worked together as a well-coordinated team.

2. Team members treated one another with respect.

3. Situational awareness was maintained (for example task prioritization and awareness of red flag issues).

4. Important issues were well communicated at hand-offs, such as during shift changes and patient transfers.

5. Disagreements were openly discussed until resolved in the patient's best interest.

Behaviors specific to good teamwork are evaluated by asking observers to rate the following:

1. Briefing and rebriefing

2. Sharing information

3. Asking for information

4. Assertion and challenge

5. Structured communication, such as SBAR

6. Closing the loop

7. Debriefing

Three essential leadership behaviors amenable to observation are as follows:

1. Leadership invited the input/feedback of others.

2. Leadership directed the team through its tasks.

3. Leadership managed conflict.

The 21 observable components are defined on the back of the metrics sheet, and observers are instructed to read the definitions prior to every observation to help ensure consistency in grading similar events.

As previously mentioned, careful collection of observed information is only the first part of turning observations into useful data. The presentation of the material is key to understanding and applying the findings to change and improvement. Two aspects of observation data stand out. First is how frequently the 21 components are seen compared to the observers' expectations that they be seen. Second, when the behaviors are viewed, what is their quality? The most recent graphing of the data shows both components. (*See* Figure 7-1 on page 66.)

Figure 7-1. Frequency and Quality of Observations

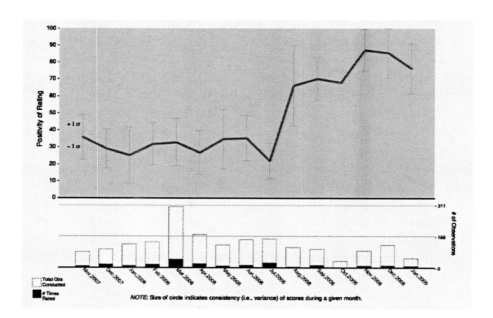

This figure presents a sample page displaying trendlines for the Behaviors Domain and includes how frequently behaviors were seen (the bars on the bottom) and the overall quality of the behaviors in the trendline.

Source: Pascal Metrics, Inc. Used with permission.

The CATS Model

Variations of the Communication and Teamwork Skills (CATS) observation tool are in use in organizations around the country. Recently, researchers at Partners Health Care developed a behavioral observation tool, based on principles of crisis resource management in nonmedical industries, which is designed to quantitatively assess communication and team skills of health care providers in a variety of real and simulated clinical settings.[7] Within this tool, specific behavior markers used for observation are clustered into the following four categories:

1. Coordination
2. Cooperation
3. Situational awareness
4. Communication

These four domains are subdivided into various elements, including the following:

- Planning and preparation
- Prioritization
- Execution
- Identifying and using resources
- Coordinating team activities
- Communicating and exchanging information
- Assertiveness and authority
- Assessing capabilities
- Supporting others
- Gathering information
- Understanding and recognition
- Anticipation
- Identifying options
- Balancing risks and selecting options
- Reevaluation

Teams are scored in terms of the occurrence and quality of specific behaviors during a routine or critical event. The

Figure 7-2. CATS Observation Form

Category	Behaviors	Observed and Good	Variation in Quality	Expected but Not Observed
Coordination	Briefing			
	Verbalize plan			
	Verbalize expected time frames			
	Debriefing			
Awareness	Visually scan environment			
	Verbalize adjustments in plan as changes occur			
Cooperation	Request external resources if needed			
	Ask for help from team as needed			
	Verbally request team input			
	Cross Monitoring			
	Verbal assertion			
	Receptive to assertion and ideas			
Communication	Closed loop			
	SBAR			
	Verbal updates—think aloud			
	Use names			
	Communicate with patient			
	Appropriate tone of voice			

This scoring sheet is used to document the performance of observed behaviors.

Source: Partners Health Care, Inc. Used with permission.

scoring sheet (*see* Figure 7-2, above) is designed to allow the observer to mark each time that specific behaviors (*see* Sidebar 7-1 on page 68) occur and grade their quality. Three columns are provided for this:

1. "Observed and Good"

2. "Variation in Quality" (meaning incomplete or of variable quality)

3. "Expected but Not Observed"

Observers score behaviors on the degree to which the behavior meets a previously agreed upon definition.

After each behavior is scored, a weighted total is obtained as follows:

- Marks in the "Observed and Good" column = 1
- Marks in the "Variation in Quality" column = .5
- Marks in the "Expected but not Observed" column = 0

Scores are added together to achieve a weighted total. Thereafter, a second total is obtained by simply adding up the total number of marks made. The weighted total, divided by the total number of marks, adjusted to a 100-point scale, is the quality score for that behavior. In this manner, a quality score is established for each behavior during each observation period. Organizations using the CATS tool can then graphically display the different scores to show the current picture of teamwork, a comparison between pre-training and post-training teams, and areas of improvement.

No matter which method of direct observation you use, measuring teamwork with a systematic process involving trained observers monitoring predefined team behaviors can help your organization get a realistic picture of how teamwork and communication occurs on a particular unit.

Sidebar 7-1. Behaviors Observed Using the CATS Tool

Following are the types of behaviors observed using the CATS tool. Three behaviors were identified as not consistently applicable in routine, noncrisis situations—"establishing an event manager," "escalation of asserted concern," and "critical language." These behaviors were positioned at the bottom of the CATS tool for use during critical events or if a routine event became critical.

- *Briefing*: As discussed in Chapter 6, this is a conversation and two-way dialogue of concise and relevant information shared prior to a procedure or activity.

- *Verbalize plan*: Speak aloud the next steps for the procedure and/or care of the patient.

- *Verbalize expected time frames*: Speak aloud time frames for particular interventions. "We'll give this another two minutes and if there's no change we'll try X."

- *Debriefing*: A conversation and two-way dialogue of concise and relevant information shared after the procedure or activity is completed.

- *Establish event manager if crisis arises*: Verbally identify who's in charge if situation becomes a crisis; event manager does not participate in active interventions but maintains situational awareness and verbalizes plans, needs, and time frames.

- *Visually scan environment*: Clinicians look up, look at one another, look at equipment, and look around the room.

- *Verbalize adjustments in plan as changes occur*: Speak aloud new plans, changes in strategy or intervention, and new time lines as procedure progresses.

- *Request additional external resources if needed*: Speak aloud, asking for help from outside the team—other clinicians, rooms, equipment, consults, and so forth.

- *Ask for help from team as needed*: Team members speak aloud, asking for assistance from members of the team.

- *Verbally request team input*: Ask aloud for team's suggestions, opinions, comments, or ideas.

- *Cross-monitoring*: Acknowledge concerns of others—watching team members, awareness of their actions, verbally stating concerns, sharing workload, verbally updating others in a manner less formal than briefing, responding to the concerns of team members.

- *Speak up, verbal assertion:* If team members are uncomfortable or unclear, they speak aloud their concerns and state an alternative viewpoint or suggest an alternative course of action. Individuals are sufficiently persistent to clearly state their opinions. If team members perceive something as unsafe, they speak aloud to indicate that. If responses to expressed concerns are not satisfactory and unsafe situations continue, individuals escalate the concern by bringing in other clinicians.

- *Closed-loop communication*: When a request is made of team members, someone specifically affirms aloud that they will complete the task and states aloud when the task has been completed.

- *SBAR:* Use of specific structured communication that states the situation, background, assessment, and recommendation.

- *Critical language*: Use of key phrases understood by all team members to mean "stop and listen; we have a potential problem." Specific phrases may differ from one institution or work unit to another.

- *Verbal updates of situation*: Think aloud—Team members verbally state their perceptions, actions, and plans as the procedure progresses.

- *Use team members' names*: Use team members' names.

- *Communicate with patient*: Team members speak to and respond to the patient

- *Use appropriate tone of voice*: Team members use a tone of voice that is calm, professional, and not unnecessarily loud.

Source: Frankel A., et al.: Using the communication and teamwork skills (CATS) assessment to measure health care team performance. *Jt Comm J Qual Patient Saf* 33:549–558, Sep. 2007.

REFERENCES

1. Yule S.: Surgeons' non-technical skills in the operating room: Reliability testing of the NOTSS behavior rating system. *World J Surg* 32:548–556, Apr. 2008.

2. Rodriguez-Paz J.M., Pronovost P.J.: Prevention of catheter-related bloodstream infections. *Adv Surg* 42:229–248, 2008.

3. Mazzocco K., et al.: Surgical team behaviors and patient outcomes. *The Am J Surg* Sep. 11, 2008.

4. Garvin D.A., Edmondson A.C., Gino F.: Is yours a learning organization? *Harv Bus Rev* 86:109–116, 134, 2008.

5. Groff H., Martin P.B. (eds.): Understanding CRICO's perinatal claims. *Forum* 21:1–14, Mar. 2001.

6. The Joint Commission: *Sentinel Event Alert 30.* http://www.jointcommission.org/SentinelEvents/SentinelEventAlert/sea_30.htm (last accessed Nov. 9, 2007).

7. Frankel A., Gardner R., Maynard L.: Using the communication and teamwork skills (CATS) assessment to measure health care team performance. *Jt Comm J Qual Patient Saf* 33:549–558, Sep. 2007.

Chapter Eight

DISCLOSURE

Doug Bonacum, Annie Herlik, and Michael Leonard

Despite the best of intentions and highly skilled caregivers, sometimes patients suffer inadvertent harm. A surgeon unintentionally nicks a patient's liver during a procedure. A patient has an unexpected heart attack during surgery. A patient is seriously injured after receiving the wrong dose of medication. Due to a mix-up in drawing lab specimens, a patient receives the wrong blood and has a fatal transfusion reaction. All these events are considered unanticipated, and every hospital in the country experiences them.

An unanticipated outcome can be caused by many things including the following[1]:

- Inherent risks associated with an intervention
- Biologic variability—the confluence of rare and unavoidable circumstances
- The patient's condition
- Human error, either an act of omission or commission
- Issues associated with clinical processes and treatment
- Malfunctions in a system used to provide care

While the previous chapters introduce the concept of systematically reducing risk and preventing errors from happening or preventing them from harming the patient, this chapter focuses on what to do when a medical error or other unanticipated event causes patient harm. Though the process of disclosure is similar in the two scenarios, they are very different dynamics: one where avoidable harm occurred related to the failure to deliver appropriate care; the latter in which unanticipated events, either related to the patient's biologic variability or the care process led to an undesired outcome. In addition to learning from the error or adverse event, organizations must be open and honest about what happened with patients, family, and the staff members involved. The process of telling the patient and family honestly what happened, how it happened, and what's going to happen next is called disclosure.

DISCLOSING ADVERSE EVENTS

Traditionally, health care organizations have shied away from disclosing adverse events to patients and their families for fear of lawsuits, inflammatory media reports, and bad publicity. According to one study by Wu et al., two thirds of residents in training surveyed admitted making a serious mistake, and yet only 50% disclosed that mistake to the attending physician, and only 25% of errors were disclosed to the patient.[2] In addition to being afraid, providers who are involved with a medical mistake bring feelings of guilt, anxiety, and shame to the situation. All of these do not easily lend themselves to open and honest disclosure.

There are four main reasons why disclosing an adverse event is important:

1. It is the right thing to do. Patients and their families have a fundamental right to know what happened, how it happened, and how it can be prevented for the next patient. Consider if it were your family member. Wouldn't you want them to know what happened?

2. An adverse event has a huge lasting impact on everyone involved, and disclosure helps participants initiate the coping process. Open communication about an error helps patients and their families to understand why all outcomes cannot be anticipated and can reduce the patient and family's anger and frustration. This is essential to help rebuild trust. In addition, openly communicating about the situation may help a provider learn from the event and maintain a sense of personal and professional integrity. We often neglect the reality that health professionals are frequently the "second victim" of an adverse event.[3] Effective disclosure is an opportunity to reaffirm and build upon the existing relationship between the people providing care and the patient and family.

3. By communicating openly about errors with patients and their families as well as with staff you can identify and repair system issues that led to the error and identify oppor-

tunities for improvement.

4. If you carry out the disclosure process well, recent evidence has shown you can actually reduce the risk of litigation and improve the public's perception of your organization. (*See* Sidebar 8-1, right.) This can be clearly seen at the University of Michigan, where highly effective patient-professional communication takes place in response to disappointing outcomes, internal error reporting has increased fivefold since 2001, and claims have decreased by 80%.[4]

Overcoming the Fear of Litigation

When establishing strong commitment to and a process for disclosure, one of the most significant barriers your organization will need to overcome is the fear of being sued. Although there is evidence that suggests if you are open and honest with people around disclosure, you decrease the risk of malpractice, some providers are still hesitant. The fact is that people sue because there is a significant divergence between expectations and outcomes, and organizations don't manage that divergence effectively.[5–7] Given that the natural emotion associated with a bad outcome and inadequate disclosure/communication is anger, anger and a goal to hurt the hospital or physician is typically the driving force toward litigation. It naturally follows then that providers who communicate openly, honestly, empathetically, and in a timely manner about the differences between expectations and outcomes will help reduce the likelihood of being sued. (*See* Sidebar 8-2 on page 71.)

Consider the following two examples. Several years ago, Abington Memorial Hospital—a 570-bed regional teaching hospital located in eastern Pennsylvania—treated an elderly gentleman, and, through a series of unfortunate diagnostic errors, inadvertently contributed to his death. Within the organization's quality assurance process, Abington discovered the error and determined that, although the family never questioned their loved one's death, the hospital felt obligated to disclose the missteps, which resulted in contributing to his untimely demise.

The treating physician and leaders from the organization visited the widow at her home and explained what happened, how it happened, and how very sorry they were. The patient's wife appreciated the organization's candor and responded by donating money to the organization to establish a memorial lectureship series in her husband's name at the hospital devoted to

---

safety. Within this series, patient safety experts from around the country come to the hospital and speak about preventing error, creating a just culture, requiring open disclosure, and improving the quality and safety of the care they deliver. This also positively reinforces the prevailing safety culture of the hospital.

On the other side of the country is a well-respected institution in which a 9-year-old girl with a highly curable form of acute leukemia entered the hospital for treatment. While in the hospital she developed a serious infection, which was not appropriately detected, and she died an avoidable death. Little explanation was provided to the family, and the organization has avoided the mother's pleas for information, despite multiple promises.

What does it say to this devastated family when they walk on the floor of the hospital where their child was a patient and no one will "look them in the eye"? The family, who went home without their child, will never be the same, and feels a profound lack of resolution and affirmation of their loss. The organization has clinicians who have been emotionally scarred by their involvement, and there is no open forum for learning, grieving, and improvement. The resident in charge of the girl's care was so upset that she quit her job.

Despite multiple interactions, the family does not believe that they have had the "right conversation" with the hospital. What does the family want—the truth, an apology, and someone to acknowledge there were lapses in care, and discuss what the organization has learned and done to prevent this tragic event from happening again? Nobody wins in this dynamic.

Sidebar 8-2. The COPIC Program

One of the best-known private-sector disclosure programs is the "3Rs" (Recognize–Respond–Resolve) program at COPIC, a liability insurer directed by physicians in Colorado. COPIC insures approximately 6,000 physicians and is the largest insurer in Colorado. In 2000 the company developed the 3Rs program, which is designed to facilitate transparent communication about injuries and expedite limited compensation—up to $30,000 per patient—for out-of-pocket health care expenses and "loss of time, and other expenses incurred as a result of a new disability, extended rehabilitation or increased care." COPIC worked with Colorado legislators so the program is "no-fault" in that it does not tie compensation to evidence of fault on the provider's part. The payments are not made in response to written demands after patients are informed of the program, and patients do not waive their rights to sue.

In its tenure, the 3Rs program has handled more than 3,000 events; approximately one quarter of the patients involved received payments averaging $5,400 each. Only seven patients who received requested payments decided to pursue litigation, and only two cases resulted in additional tort payments. Although the range of cases handled by the COPIC program is limited, the outcomes suggest that many adverse events can be resolved without litigation. In addition, the low average payment per incident reinforces the notion that patients are looking for help with real aspects of their situation—a plane ticket so their mother can fly in to help take care of the kids, money for the truck payment, or supplemental childcare—and are not trying to capitalize on the situation.[8]

LEADERSHIP COMMITMENT TO DISCLOSURE IS CRITICAL

As mentioned in Chapter 1, an effective approach to disclosure cannot exist without significant and visible leadership support. To realize such an approach, organization leadership must do following:

- Model organization values in times that are difficult. Disclosure conversations are never easy, and yet they are a clear sign of how much an organization's values are imbedded in the way it does business. Disclosure represents a true test of a culture in that it shows that the organization does the right thing even when it's not easy. The ability and willingness to do this sends important messages to the community and internally within the organization.

- Commit to a fair and just culture. (*See* Chapter 3 for more information.) Effective disclosure is dependent on a just culture. If a provider doesn't feel safe about speaking up about errors, there is no way they will be comfortable sharing information with a patient.

- Be actively engaged in learning about adverse and potentially compensable events. What percentage of lawsuits and demand letters are you actively aware of and managing? The answer should be close to 100%; in many care systems it is only 30%, making it difficult to resolve issues early.

- Design and implement a systematic approach/structure on how to disclose unexpected outcomes to patients and families. Effective disclosure needs to be done in a systematic and consistent fashion. Structure and ownership for the process are essential. Organizations must have a systematic way that disclosure conversations occur, and such a process must be created with input from multiple disciplines, including administrative leaders, medical staff leaders, attorneys, patient safety professionals, and risk managers. Such a process needs to involve designated individuals—such as a Healthcare Ombudsman Mediator (HCOM), situation management team, or other type of mediator—who drive the process. More about the HCOM program is provided below, beginning on page 74.

- Provide regular education for providers about the importance of effective communication and how to partner with patients to achieve safe care. Effective communication begins the moment a patient enters a health care facility and meets his or her physicians. By taking the time to explain options, listen to concerns, communicate with sincerity, be humble about their abilities, and realistic about the risks and uncertainties inherent in health care, providers set the tone for collaboration and trust. If the patient perceives a provider as helpful, communicative, and honest, the patient will have more understanding in a situation where things get out of control. Conversely, if a patient perceives a provider as removed, aloof, short-tempered, and condescending, the patient is more likely to blame the provider when a situation ends poorly. Poor relationships with physicians translate directly to lawsuits. Patients who perceive the patient-provider relationship as respectful often refuse to sue the provider; however, if the patient believes the relationship is not respectful, there can be a strong desire to name the provider in the lawsuit whether he or she is culpable or not.

The central conclusion of a recent study by Hickson et al. is that the inability to establish rapport with the patient is a root cause of increased risk of malpractice suits. This research shows that 6% of doctors attract 40% of lawsuits and generate 85% of malpractice losses.[9] In another study by Ambady et al., the tone of the surgeon's voice alone was linked to future malpractice claims. Four 10-second segments of the surgeon's voice were recorded at the beginning and end of patient meetings. The recordings were scrambled so that the researchers could hear only the surgeon's tone of voice. Based on listening to the tone of the surgeon's voice for 40 seconds, college students could predict 85% of the time the malpractice history of the physician.[10]

To achieve significant change in a provider's communication style, didactic lectures are not sufficient. When educating providers on improving communication, it is very helpful to use real scenarios in which providers can be debriefed for personal improvement. As previously mentioned, this not only provides procedural learning—"I have done this and know how"—but also helps people become more comfortable with inherently difficult conversations. From a strategic perspective, it may be useful to have the goals of broadly enhancing communication between caregivers and patients related to plans, risks, day-to-day outcomes, and informed consent. In addition, having "just in time" training and support related to disclosing major adverse events is essential.

HOW TO DISCLOSE

As a first step to disclosure, organizations need leadership commitment that open, honest disclosure is a basic component of the organizational culture. Policies should be developed that support and inform situations in which disclosure is needed. The Joint Commission requires such a policy to aid in the communication about and coordination of unanticipated events and serve as a template to ensure consistency and eliminate confusion when dealing with an adverse event. The policy should be created with input from a multidisciplinary group, including physicians, nurses, risk managers, patient safety officers, and senior leadership. Such a plan should include the following elements:

• Objectives and principles of the disclosure process. This could include the need to be honest, compassionate, and understanding in communications with patients.

• A description of the type of events that will trigger the plan

• Roles and responsibilities of health care staff and organization leadership

• Reporting process and timelines

• Checklists to help with event management

• Development of the situation management team.

Despite having an established process for disclosure, every adverse event is different, and the specifics of the process will vary depending on what happened, the players involved, and the nature of the outcomes. To help navigate the disclosure process, organizations may want to create a situation management team. This is a multidisciplinary group that comes together to best address the nuances involved in a particular case and provide direction and support to the individuals directly working with the patients and families. Depending on the specific organization, the individuals that make up this team will vary, however core team members could include the following:

—Risk manager

—Hospital leadership

—Physician leader

—Nursing leader

—Ethicist

—The ombudsman or other designated mediator—some organizations keep the ombudsman out of this process so he or she can preserve "neutrality" in his or her dealings with the patient, family, and caregivers.

—In specific situations, it may be helpful to include others on the situation management team, such as the department head of the area in which the event occurred, the provider, a representative from public relations, or others involved in the event.[1]

Some other things to keep in mind when developing the policy is that when things go wrong, there are three things that patients most want:

• An honest explanation as to what happened

• An empathetic statement or apology related to the unanticipated outcome, demonstrating that the organization cares what happened to their loved one

• Information about what the organization is doing and will do to fix the problem so it won't happen to anyone else

Within the plan, organizations may also want to outline a step-by-step process that providers can use to ensure appropriate and timely disclosure. Although there are no hard and fast rules on how to effectively disclose information and solicit ideas or requests from patients to aid in the resolution of their event, following is one effective approach. When a major unanticipated event occurs do the following:

1. Stabilize the patient.

2. Treat any injury.

3. Prevent further harm.

4. Eliminate any obvious remaining threat to patient safety, such as an impaired provider, faulty equipment, an unsafe system of care, or a seriously deficient protocol.

5. Immediately secure implicated drugs, equipment, and records.

6. Document all actions in the medical record.

7. If the primary provider is impaired, immediately provide a substitute and inform the patient and family.

8. Ensure that all members of the care team are fully aware of the issues so that subsequent communication with the patient and family is consistent.

9. Engage risk management professionals.

10. Establish who will have primary responsibility for communicating with the patient and family about the event. This may be the physician or provider involved in the event, an ombudsman, a member of the situation management team, the risk manager, or the patient safety officer.

11. Communicate with the patient and family about the event. As soon as possible, the patient and family should learn of the event and the facts as known. Delay for the purpose of a more thorough disclosure is typically counterproductive, especially if it is apparent that something is wrong. All communication regarding an event should involve an objective description of the event, its consequences, and the processes being used to analyze and review systems in order to minimize the chances of the event recurring. There should also be ample opportunity for questions from the family.

12. Let the patient and family know what future communication they can expect and make it clear there will be many conversations and that they will continue until the patient and family are satisfied.

During the disclosure, staff should refrain from offering subjective information, speculation, or beliefs relating to possible causes of the adverse event, as that can further confuse the situation and lead to possible liability. It is absolutely acceptable to say, "Here is what we know right now; there are some things we need to look at more closely and learn about, and when we have done this we will come back and tell you." Staff must absolutely refrain from offering comments or criticisms of the health care team.

While every effort should be made to help the patient and family, staff should not promise what cannot be delivered. This will only lead to frustration and anger on the part of the patient and family. (*See* Sidebars 8-3, 8-4, and 8-5 on pages 74–75 for further suggestions on the content, tone, and structure of the disclosure conversation.)

13. Provide access to emotional and psychological support for the patient and family as long as it is required.

14. Support the patient care team. A fundamental element involved in disclosure is leadership support for practitioners and spokespersons. Providers should not be made to feel guilty as a result of an unanticipated adverse event but, on the contrary, should feel strongly supported and valued. Physicians and other health care personnel will generally need some form of emotional support in the aftermath of a major untoward event, particularly if it involved an error. In the management plan, organizations should identify individuals or departments that can provide this type of support. Regarding the event itself, staff members should be provided as much information as possible and told what they can discuss and with whom. Any promises made to staff should be fulfilled.

15. Determine the circumstances surrounding the event and the contributing factors as quickly as possible while memories of those involved are fresh.

16. Report the error to the appropriate parties. Depending on the error, different departments, entities, or agencies may need to be notified. For example, the risk manager, patient safety officer, or quality improvement department may need to be notified.

17. As soon as practical, all involved parties should participate in a systematic analysis of the event. Generally, root cause analyses are reserved for sentinel events. Although adverse events are difficult and painful for all involved, they do present a unique opportunity for learning. As previously discussed, organizations should carefully review the circumstances behind events and look for underlying system failures that can be addressed in order to prevent further error.

18. In follow-up meetings with the family and patient, appropriate staff should communicate the results of the analysis and corrective action plans

Who Should Disclose?

Disclosure is a trained skill, and one that does not come

Sidebar 8-3. Guiding Principle of the Disclosure Conversation

After providing known facts of the event, consider the following guiding principles to enhance communication with patients and families during disclosure and subsequent conversations:

- Give the patient and/or patient's representative immediate and ample time to discuss the event.
- Use active listening skills, including solid eye contact, open posture, and empathetic listening.
- Be sensitive to cultural differences and the need for interpretative services.
- Correct false statements or impressions factually without being defensive.
- Address any misunderstandings, confusion, or information gaps.
- Give the patient and/or patient's representative an honest response to his or her questions, including the fact that you may not be able to answer all of the questions. If there is another individual within the organization to whom you can refer the patient, you should inform the patient of this option.
- Proactively initiate subsequent communications.
- Deliver what you promise.
- Follow a statement about information that will be held confidential with, *"But what we can tell you is. . ."*

It is also known that a very common problem with professionals who feel guilty or worried is they often communicate more than is useful. Practice sessions can be very helpful prior to difficult conversations.

Source: Communicating Unanticipated Adverse Events Program, Kaiser Permanente. Used with permission.

Sidebar 8-4. Watch Your Tone

When communicating with a patient, health care providers should be aware of their tone of voice (is it measured and calm?), the pace of the conversation (are pauses long enough to allow those receiving the information to take in what has just been said?), and the power of touch and a direct gaze. Within the conversation, the speaker should give the impression that he or she has all the time needed to have this important conversation. Body language can speak volumes and make all the difference in the way patients and their families respond to what health care providers have to say.

THE BENEFITS OF A HEALTH CARE OMBUDSMAN PROGRAM (HCOM)

One approach to designating individuals for disclosure is to create an HCOM program. An ombudsman participates in disclosure conversations with patients and families, works to resolve issues and answer questions associated with an event, and acts as a go-between for the organization and the patient and family. An ombudsman functions independently of the organization and reports directly to the CEO or other senior leader. Neither an advocate for the patient nor for the institution, the ombudsman is an advocate for a fair process. He or she interviews all participants in an event to try to get answers for the patient. He or she also works with the patient and family to determine their needs regarding the situation. Confidentiality is maintained, and information shared in confidence with the ombudsman is not disclosed, similar to the confidentiality required of a mediator.

The following hypothetical example shows one way an ombudsman program can be used.

During Mr. Jones's hand surgery, the surgeon operates on the wrong hand. As soon as the surgeon realizes the error, he contacts the ombudsman, who comes to the operating room. After the patient is stabilized, the surgeon talks to the ombudsman about what happened. The ombudsman then convenes the situation management team.

The situation management team talks about the event and determines what is known, what can be shared immediately with the patient and family, what needs to be further investigated, who should communicate with the patient and family, and who will do the investigation. The group also discusses the best methods for communicating with the patient and family.

---

naturally to most people. Ideally, all health care training should include effective communication and disclosure skills. In organizations delivering care, actually training everyone is a huge task. In addition, a provider who has been a part of an incident may not be in a position to effectively communicate with the patient and family, and an impartial perspective may be beneficial.

To address these issues, you may want to consider the model where you train a few individuals to become "experts" in disclosure. These individuals come on site when there is a disclosure situation to aid the physician and facilitate direct communication with staff, the patient, and his or her family. These individuals should be trained and given the tools to have effective conversations. They should be compassionate individuals with excellent communication skills who are able to look at a situation from multiple vantage points.

Sidebar 8-5. The SPIKES Protocol

A strategy for communicating bad news, called the SPIKES protocol, may be helpful in disclosure conversations. This protocol highlights the most important features of a bad news interview and suggests methods of assessing the situation as it evolves and responding constructively to what happens. Following is a brief description of the steps within the protocol:

Setting (S)

This involves considering the appropriate environment for the discussion. One aspect of the environment would be the location. Such a location should be appropriate for a sensitive, private, and potentially devastating discussion. Ideally, this could be an interview room, an office with the door closed, or curtains drawn around a hospital bed. Within the setting, distractions—such as the radio or television—should be eliminated.

In addition to location, providers should consider involving significant others as appropriate to give the patient some support. The provider should look attentive and calm during the interview, be sitting down, maintain eye contact, and use active listening skills to communicate caring. Repeating back what the patient communicated may also convey how much the provider is listing.

Providers should be fully present in the conversation. Before an important discussion, they should make arrangements for the phones to be answered by other staff members or voice mail and make sure that other staff members do not interrupt the meeting. If phone calls or other interruptions do occur, providers should courteously address them so that the patient doesn't feel less important than the interruption.

Perception (P)

Before a provider breaks bad news to a patient, he or she should glean a fairly accurate picture of their perception of the medical situation—in particular, how they view the seriousness of the condition. Some questions to ask may be "What have you been told about all this so far?" and "Are you worried that this might be something serious?"

Invitation (I)

This is the time in which you try to assess how much information the patient or family would like. Some patients do not want to know all the details of their medical situation while others want to know everything. Based on the answer to this question, a provider can gauge how much detail to give. This step should not be confused with determining how much of the truth to tell the patient and family, but more how much detail about the truth to give. For example, some patients may just want to know that the wrong hand has been operated on, why it happened, and the consequences of the problem, while others may want to know more details of the situation.

Knowledge (K)

Before you break bad news, give the patient a warning that bad news is coming. There's no need for the provider to drop a bombshell when he or she can ease into the topic. This gives the patient and family a few seconds longer to prepare psychologically for the bad news. Examples of warning statements include, "Unfortunately, I've got some bad news to tell you, Mr. Andrews." or "Mrs. Smith, I'm so sorry to have to tell you. . ."

It is also helpful to give the information in small chunks and clarify patient understanding at the end of each chunk. For example, use the phrases "Do you see what I mean?" or "Is this making sense so far?" Given issues around health literacy and the stress of these situations, using a "teach-back" technique is important. For example, "can you please tell me how you'll describe our conversation to the rest of your family?"

Empathy (E)

Responding to patients' emotions is one of the most difficult parts of breaking bad news. Within a disclosure conversation, it is important to acknowledge patients' emotions as they arise and to address them. A helpful technique in this process is "the empathetic response," and it is made up of three straightforward steps:

Step 1: Listen for and identify the emotion (or mixture of emotions).

Step 2: Identify the cause or source of the emotion, which is most likely to be the bad news that the patient has just heard.

Step 3: Show your patient that you have made the connection between the above two steps—that is, that you have identified the emotion and its origin.

After you have identified the emotion and origin it is important to validate the patient's feelings. It may be helpful to use phrases such as "I can understand how you can feel that way." By empathizing and validating, a provider can relate that he or she understands the human side to the medical issue or event and can relate to the patient's feelings.

Strategy and Summary (S)

Before the discussion ends, it is helpful to summarize the information in the discussion and give the patient an opportunity to voice any major concerns or questions.[11]

When the situation management team meets, the ombudsman and the surgeon meet with the family. The surgeon and ombudsman take the family to a private location to discuss the situation. They engage in a compassionate and honest conversation with the family, explaining what happened, what is occurring right now, and what is still not known. During the conversation, both the ombudsman and the surgeon are careful to communicate the facts that are known at the time, rather than conjecture, and make sure their explanations are understandable and empathetic.

They also discuss how they are going to continue to care for the patient and what he should expect. In this case, the surgeon offers to continue providing care—the patient still needs the intended surgery—and also offers the option of another surgeon taking over the care if that is the patient's preference. There is also a conversation about what steps will be taken to rectify the situation, as in a waiver of fees or other appropriate measures.

After the initial conversation takes place, the surgeon returns to his work while the ombudsman remains with the family to further answer any questions and identify any logistical needs the family might have. The ombudsman works to meet the immediate needs of the family and identifies any additional information that is necessary.

When the family understands the situation, the ombudsman leaves the family and updates the situation manage- ment team. The ombudsman remains in close contact with the family, following up regularly to ensure that they have no further questions. Often, the first meeting is pretty shocking, and the family doesn't have time to develop questions. Sometimes they don't even hear everything that is said. That is why it is important to contact them later to follow up on questions and ensure that they are aware of what is going on.

After the initial disclosure conversation, the organization works to investigate the event. As a result of this investigation, the organization puts protocols in place and educates the staff on these protocols to prevent such an event from happening again. The surgeon and ombudsman meet with the patient and family, take responsibility for the event, and offer an apology. They show the patient the protocols that have been put in place and also share information about the education provided to the staff on preventing wrong-site surgeries.

While Mr. Jones is frustrated about the operation, he appreciates the organization's candor and apology and is pleased it has implemented systems to prevent the event from happening to someone else. Mr. Jones and his family express gratitude for the organization's honesty and compassion. Mr. Jones and the surgeon shake hands.

Who Makes a Good Ombudsman

The ideal ombudsman has strong interpersonal skills, understands medical terminology and medical records, knows the organizational structure of the organization, and is respected by the providers who ultimately must place their trust in him or her. The key skill necessary for an effective ombudsman is communication. The ombudsman relies heavily on shuttle diplomacy, problem solving, and interpersonal communication skills. He or she should receive significant training in mediation and ombudsman skills, participate in one-on-one coaching for a period of time while establishing his or her position within the health care setting, and participate in regularly scheduled reflective practice and advanced trainings to further develop his or her conflict resolution and communication skills. Kaiser Permanente has extensive experience with this concept, having implemented their HCOM program in more than 30 hospitals. The authors are happy to share information about the collective experience.

In conclusion, effective disclosure is very difficult and takes great skill. Being involved in a situation where a patient has experienced avoidable harm pushes every button clinicians have with regard to whether they are competent, were paying enough attention, and were trying hard enough. Such situations are often seriously threatening to their sense of self-esteem, as they have all been taught repeatedly that "good doctors and nurses don't make mistakes," and now they are dealing with one on a profound level.

When we deal with patients and their families in these very difficult and delicate situations, we need to do something that feels vulnerable and threatening—openly engage the patient and his or her family, even if they are angry and frustrated. All too often, we back off, and the patient perceives neglect and abandonment in the setting in which he or she were harmed.

Effective disclosure requires structure, skill, and organizational commitment. The benefit is that it offers great value to patients and families as well as clinicians and the organization as a whole.

REFERENCES

1. Leonard M., Frankel A., Simmonds T.: *Achieving Safe and Reliable healthcare.* Chicago: Health Administration Press, 2004.

2. Wu A.W., et al.: Do house officers learn from their mistakes? *JAMA* 265:2089–2094, 1991.

3. Wu A.W.: Medical error: The second victim. *BMJ* 320:726–727, Mar. 18, 2000.

4. Boothman R.: Testimony before the United States Senate, Committee on Health, Education, Labor and Pensions, Jun. 22, 2006. http://help.senate.gov/Hearings/2006_06_22/boothman.pdf.

5. Hickson G.B., et al.: Factors that prompted families to file medical malpractice claims following perinatal injuries. *JAMA* 267:1359–1363, Mar. 11, 1992.

6. Wu A.W.: Handling hospital errors: Is disclosure the best defense? *Ann Intern Med* 131:970–972, Dec. 21, 1999.

7. Kraman S.S., Hamm G.: Risk management: Extreme honesty may be the best policy, *Ann Intern Med* 131:963–967, Dec. 21, 1999.

8. Gallagher T.H., Studdert D., Levinson W.: Disclosing harmful medical errors to patients. *N Engl J Med* 356:2713, Jun. 28, 2007.

9. Hickson G.B., et al.: Patient complaints and malpractice risk. *JAMA* 287:2951–2957, Jun. 12, 2002.

10. Ambady N., et al.: Surgeon's tone of voice: A clue to malpractice history. *Surgery* 132:5–9, Jul. 2002.

11. Adapted from Buckman R.A.: Breaking bad news: the S-P-I-K-E-S strategy. *Community Oncology* 2:138–142, 2005.

Chapter Nine

ENSURING PATIENT INVOLVEMENT

Gail Nielsen, Maureen Connor, Mary Ann Abrams, **and** *Michael Leonard*

As discussed in Chapter 6, teamwork is a critical component in providing safe and reliable care. Patient care teams must work collaboratively together, respect each other's input, and communicate effectively in order to ensure that the right care is given at the right time to the right patient.[1]

A key member of the patient care team is the patient. Organizations with a reliable and safe culture center medical care around the patient, empower patients to participate in their care, and actively work to include patient perspectives in improvement. Such organizations partner with patients, gather feedback about their care experiences, and solicit their input regarding the type of care they want.

The Internet and the mainstream media, among many other factors, have led to an ever increasingly well-informed patient who has specific expectations for his or her health care experience. Patients are often very aware when care doesn't go well and can provide a unique insight into an organization's processes and procedures.

Health care organizations cannot afford to ignore this essential resource. Organizations that create opportunities for patients, families, and staff to work together can improve the safety and quality of the care experience. One of the 2009 National Patient Safety Goals from The Joint Commission is specifically targeted to this topic and requires organizations to encourage patients' active involvement in their own care as a patient safety strategy.[2]

Involving patients in their care has many benefits, including the following:

- Ensures the most appropriate care for the patient
- Respects any specific cultural or emotional needs
- Potentially improves patient outcomes
- Helps identify potential system issues or gaps in care
- Helps improve staff satisfaction

Despite its many benefits, involving patients and families in their care conflicts with an old but still present philosophy of the physician as the individual provider and the patient as the recipient, not participant, in his or her care. Achieving a culture centered on the patient takes bold leadership. Leadership must embrace the concept of patient and family inclusion, promote it among staff and patients, and invest in resources and training to build the collaborative skills of staff.

WAYS TO INVOLVE PATIENTS

There are many ways to involve patients in the care delivery process. The following sections examine a few of these ways.

Involve Patients and Caregivers in Treatment Decisions

Involving patients in their treatment decisions helps individuals to understand their illness and treatment options and can also help them recognize when treatment deviates from expected. This not only respects the patient's rights and preferences, but can help organizations identify errors and point out inconsistencies. (*See* Sidebar 9-1 on page 80.) Organizations can involve patients in their care by taking some of the following steps:

- Share care plans. This can be accomplished through continuous discussion with physicians and nurses about the type of treatment a patient needs and the state of his or her recovery.

- Review daily goals sheets. A daily goal sheet outlines every goal for the patient for a particular day. These goals, which may be clinical or social in nature, are areas in which the patient needs to have significant input. An example of a clinical goal would be to have a patient off his or her ventilator by the end of the day. A social goal might be to have the patient able to watch his favorite TV show. Whatever the goals listed on the daily goal sheets, the clinicians should discuss and review them with the patient and his or her

Sidebar 9-1. Empowering Patients to Speak Up

In March 2002, The Joint Commission, together with the Centers for Medicare & Medicaid Services (CMS), launched a national campaign to urge patients to take a role in preventing health care errors by becoming active, involved, and informed participants on the health care team. The program features free, downloadable brochures, posters, and buttons on a variety of patient safety topics, including the following[4]:

- Preventing errors
- Avoiding mistakes in surgery
- Information for living organ donors
- Five things to prevent infection
- Avoiding mistakes with medicines
- Research studies
- Follow-up care
- Preventing medical test mistakes
- Patient rights
- Understanding physicians and other caregivers
- Pain management

Within each topic, the Speak Up™ campaign encourages the public to do the following:

Speak up if you have questions or concerns, and if you don't understand, ask again. It's your body and you have a right to know.

Pay attention to the care you are receiving. Make sure you're getting the right treatments and medications by the right health care professionals. Don't assume anything.

Educate yourself about your diagnosis, the medical tests you are undergoing, and your treatment plan.

Ask a trusted family member or friend to be your advocate.

Know what medications you take and why you take them. Medication errors are the most common health care mistakes.

Use a hospital, clinic, surgery center, or other type of health care organization that has undergone a rigorous on-site evaluation against established state-of-the-art quality and safety standards, such as that provided by The Joint Commission.

Participate in all decisions about your treatment. You are the center of the health care team.

discussed in Chapter 6, these are done at shift change and throughout the day so that all team members are aware of the treatment plan, daily goals, and progress toward meeting those goals.

- Involve the patient in handoffs. When a patient's care is handed off from one provider to another, it is helpful to involve the patient in the handoff process. Introducing the patient to the new provider, updating the patient on the status of achieving outcomes and goals, and reassessing the patient's feelings about those goals can all be helpful at this time. Kaiser Permanente uses a process entitled the Nurse Knowledge Exchange to involve patients in the handoff process.[3] Within this exchange, nurses hand off patient care at the bedside with the patients and family. Using a Situation, Background, Assessment, Recommendation (SBAR) format, called I-SBAR—the I standing for introduce—nurses communicate with the patient the status of his or her care and what he or she can expect during the next shift. They also introduce the nurse taking over care, so the patient can associate a face with a name. Nurses have a 60-second framing conversation before going into the patient's room to help focus the conversation and determine the two to three items on the front burner. Some units incorporate a whiteboard in the process so the nurse can write down what's going to happen, and patients and families can document any questions for the next exchange. Nurses finish the exchange by asking patients to "teach back" the material covered in the exchange. This is also a time to invite patient and family questions or correct information they believe is inaccurate. (*See* pages 84–85 for more information on the teach-back method.)

- Patients should be as involved as they want to be in their care. This means that patients should be informed about any test results, treatment plans, protocols, and procedures, as well as comprehensive education about their care that is targeted to their reading level. (*See* pages 82–87 for more information on patient education.)

Obtain and Respond to Patient and Family Feedback

As previously mentioned, the nuances of the care experience are not lost on patients. They are acutely aware of how efficient the care they receive is, how well the providers "get along," and how well they feel when leaving the facility. Organizations should tap into this wealth of opinion to help

family, and incorporate their contributions. In addition, the daily goal sheet should be posted on the patient's bed or on the door to his or her room. This way all staff associated with the patient's care can be on the same page as to what the patient's goals for treatment are.

- Involve the patient in multidisciplinary rounds. As

Sidebar 9-2. Patient and Family Councils

One specific way to involve patients is to create a patient and family council. These councils, typically made up of mostly patients and supported by health care system representatives from operations, administration, and quality, help ensure that the patient experience, point of view, and recommendations are shared in a way that creates greater respect for and profound knowledge concerning the fundamental question: "What is in the best interest of the patient?" This council can meet regularly to give input on patient care, review patient satisfaction survey results, serve as a resource for improvement initiatives throughout the organization, and initiate its own improvement projects. For example, if your department was working on a fall prevention initiative, you could solicit the patient and family council and ask for help with that project. The council could identify a liaison who would work directly with your performance improvement team.

A patient and family council can show firsthand your organization's commitment to patient involvement in care and provide a venue for patients and families to give valuable feedback in real time. Patients provide a unique perspective and when designing any new program or process, having them involved helps ensure that the process is as good as it can be. For example, before launching an initiative, your organization can test the concept with the patient and family council and receive honest, real-time feedback about the concept without having to wait three to four months for patient satisfaction survey results.

One organization that is very familiar with the concept of a patient and family council is The Dana-Farber Cancer Institute. The hospital's patient and family council has accomplished much in its 10-year existence. For instance, the group produces a newsletter written for patients and families *by* patients and families; participates in legislative activity; and helps teach other organizations how to implement patient-/family-centered programs. The hospital supplies a small budget, but all decisions in the council are made independently by the council members. Recently Dana-Farber began designing and building a new oncology and ambulatory care center. Council members were involved in the planning and helped choose the architect. Council members also participate in developing staff education materials. For example, council members were involved in creating a video on informed consent in which they gave input on how physicians can encourage patients to enroll in clinical trials and also respect patients who are not interested in being a part of clinical trials. The council also helped establish a fast track process for children with a fever and low white blood cell count in the emergency department.

The role of the patient and family council is valued at all levels of Dana-Farber. An individual cannot be hired into a senior level position without being interviewed by a member of the patient council.[5]

---

identify gaps in care and areas of opportunity. Following are some sources for patient feedback:

- Satisfaction surveys
- Focus groups
- Compliment/complaint letters
- Safety hotlines
- Staff feedback
- Community groups
- Patient and family council (*see* Sidebar 9-2, above)
- Patients as members of the patient safety and other committees

Information from these feedback sources should be analyzed and prioritized along with other issue identification and performance data. The patient safety officer plays a critical role in reviewing, analyzing, and prioritizing these data.

Partner with Patients and their Families to Improve Care Across the Organization

To truly partner with patients, you must involve them at the policy-making level. This may mean inviting them to participate on your organization's quality or safety committee, sentinel event review panel, or other performance improvement–related committee. While some organizations may balk at this idea—feeling it exposes the organization to potential lawsuits or bad press—others have embraced the concept, choosing to learn from patient perspectives and experiences rather than trying to deny them.

Consider this example. An organization was working on a new hand hygiene policy in which patients were asked to remind staff members to wash their hands. The patient representative on the committee was not comfortable with some aspects of the policy. "While it's all fine and good to ask patients to remind staff members to wash their hands," the patient said, "the ultimate responsibility for washing hands belongs to the provider, and this policy does not adequately address that." Based on the patient's feedback, the organization was able to tweak its program to emphasize provider responsibility and use patient reminders as a double check to the provider.

Patients should also be directly involved in programs that affect patients. For example, if your organization is creating a new Web site, you should seriously consider involving patients in that process. They can provide unique feedback on the site's ease of use and the appropriateness of the content and flow.

Involve Patients in Provider Education

There is no better way to educate physicians, nurses, and other direct care providers on the importance of communicating effectively with patients than to have a patient share his or her care experiences, particularly when the experiences were not positive. Providers—specifically physicians—may not be aware of how their tone, mannerisms, and bedside manner affect patients, but by listening to a patient share his or her care experience, it can swiftly and sometimes painfully be made clear.

Involve the Family Whenever Possible

Having medical procedures can be intimidating, but being separated from loved ones who can provide support makes even routine procedures more stressful. Organizations that include families in the care of patients can see improved clinical outcomes as well as increased quality of care.

Families should be part of any education provided to the patient, and they should be encouraged to participate in treatment decisions where appropriate. One way to encourage family involvement is to maintain open access to nursing units, intensive care units (ICUs), and the emergency room. By keeping these areas open to families 24 hours a day—even during shift changes, rounds, a code, and other emergency situations—you can encourage their involvement, decrease the potential for error, and increase patient safety. Along the same lines, those organizations that allow family members to stay during anesthesia induction, in the recovery room, in radiology, and during treatment and procedures open up the environment and reduce the potential for errors.[6]

ADDRESSING PATIENT LITERACY

Nearly one out of every four Americans cannot read the headlines of a newspaper and 40–44 million adults are functionally illiterate. A person who is functionally illiterate can sign his or her name and read basic information but cannot consistently understand the gist of what they read or use a tool that has many words and numbers, such as a bus schedule. He or she may be able to find an intersection on a street map or determine the difference in price on tickets but cannot consistently identify information from a bar graph or write a brief letter of complaint.

One type of literacy is health care literacy. According to Healthy People 2010, health care literacy is "the degree to which individuals have the capacity to obtain, process, and understand basic health information and services needed to make appropriate health decisions."[7] People with low health literacy can have problems with medications, appointment slips, consent forms, discharge instructions, health education materials and insurance applications. They have trouble understanding this information, following treatment plans, and seeking follow-up care, and may be unwilling or unable to ask questions.

Consider this example. Mr. Jones is a diabetic patient who recently was given instructions on how to take his insulin. Unbeknownst to his nurse, Mr. Jones cannot read. Although Mr. Jones is conscientious about taking his medicine and eating the proper foods, he is admitted to the ICU three times across three months for severe diabetic ketoacidosis, a potentially life-threatening condition. During his third admission to the ICU, the nurse, sensing something is wrong, meets with Mr. Jones and asks him to describe his diet and show how he gives himself insulin shots. Mr. Jones says that he is not able to show the nurse because he does not have an orange, and frankly, he's getting a little tired of oranges and is there any other way to administer the medication. The nurse realizes that the patient had been taught to administer insulin by injecting it into oranges, and he went home and continued to do so, eating the oranges, rather than injecting the insulin into himself! Three trips to the ICU and roughly $100,000 of cost occurred because the organization didn't get something as basic as how to administer his insulin right. Mr. Jones didn't know, and the people providing care had no idea.

People with low literacy skills are twice as likely to report their health status as poor. They tend to have lower health knowledge and less-healthy behaviors, and consequently have poorer health outcomes and greater health costs. They have a 52% greater likelihood of hospitalization, tend to use health care services more frequently than literate patients, have longer lengths of stay, and are at much higher risk for medical errors.[8–10]

How Do You Know If a Patient Has a Literacy Problem?

Low literacy is not necessarily obvious, and a patient can look and speak in a way that does not suggest a problem with health literacy. Anyone—regardless of age, race, education, or income—can have problems with health literacy. Older patients, recent immigrants, and people with chronic disease are especially vulnerable to low health literacy. People who can't read or understand health care information are usually ashamed of this fact and are very good at hiding the problem. According to one study, 70% of people who cannot read do not tell their spouse.[11] If they aren't going to tell their loved ones they can't read, what makes us think they will tell us?

Although there is no foolproof way to identify an illiterate patient, there are some telltale signs:

- It takes the patient twice as long to fill out a form.
- The patient is always "forgetting" to bring his or her glasses and asking the provider to read him or her the form.
- The patient never asks questions. Although this may be a personality trait or cultural barrier, it could also be an indication that the patient does not understand the information provided.
- You observe the patient struggling to read.
- The patient asks "where do I sign?" versus "do I sign here?"
- The patient continuously misses appointments. If your organization communicates information about the next appointment using a written appointment card, and the patient cannot read, he or she will rely on memory to keep the appointment, and as we already know, human memory is fallible.

In addition to the previously mentioned indications, low health literacy patients may bring someone who can read with them to their appointment, watch other people and do what they do, pretend they can read, or ask for help from other patients or staff. Most low-literacy patients, however, never ask for help.

Why Address Patient Literacy?

Low health literacy is not only dangerous for the patient; it costs the health care system a fortune—according to some estimates as much as $73 billion per year. Within the United States, treatments for congestive heart failure, asthma, and diabetes make up a large portion of health care

spending, and many of the individuals receiving those treatments have low literacy levels. If health care organizations designed programs to address low literacy levels among patients with these chronic conditions, the health care system could reduce the cost of health care significantly.

In addition to the financial waste, a safer health care environment is one in which patients understand what is happening to them, make *informed* health decisions, know what their role is in their care, and do not experience a sense of shame or embarrassment at any time.[12] A critical way to achieve this environment is to ensure that education provided to patients is simple, straightforward, understandable, and sensitive to cultural needs.

Make It Simple for Everyone

Some organizations believe in assessing general reading levels to help determine health literacy; however, assessing literacy levels does not ensure patient understanding in the clinical setting.[12] The best approach to educating patients is to worry less about identifying people who struggle with literacy and instead admit that low health literacy is a universal problem. If you spend a lot of time trying to separate the literate from the illiterate, you may overlook the fact that when stressed, worried, and panicking, even the most literate individuals may fail to understand complex information. All patients appreciate a simpler, easy-to-understand presentation focused on the need-to-know information. The fact is high-literacy individuals are not offended by simple clear communication.

Like so many aspects of the health care delivery process, to truly address the low literacy issue in health care organizations, you must take a systematic approach. Such an approach requires leadership support, effective tools, and comprehensive training for providers on how to educate patients and overcome literacy issues. Following are some tips organizations can use to help develop a systematic approach:

- Include the need to address health literacy in the strategic plan. This helps ensure continual resources dedicated to patient education and health literacy.
- Foster an environment in which providers communicate openly and respectfully with patients, encouraging them to speak up and be involved in their care.
- Provide a shame-free environment in which patients feel comfortable saying they don't understand, asking ques-

tions, and talking openly about their health and concerns. Organizations can achieve such an environment by encouraging staff to have an attitude of helpfulness, caring, and respect; providing easy-to-follow instructions for appointments, check-in, referrals, and tests; having simple telephone processes; providing confidential assistance; and ensuring that all staff members understand their role in enhancing patient understanding.

• Create patient-friendly education materials (*See* Sidebar 9-4 on page 85.). Written education, when done well, can be a helpful supplement to the patient-provider conversation. Often, however, such materials include complex medical terms, are written at a level above the patient's ability to understand, contain too much information, and are not designed to be easy to read. To help improve the likelihood that written materials will be effective, consider the following strategies:

—Use simple words (1–2 syllables), short sentences (4–6 words), and short paragraphs (2–3 sentences). This is sometimes called plain language. (*See* Sidebar 9-3, right.)

—Separate text with headings and bullets.

—Incorporate lots of white space.

—Avoid medical jargon.

—Prominently locate the "need-to-know" information.

—Use drawings and pictures to illustrate points. These should support the text; be simple, realistic, and culturally appropriate, and show the correct way to do things.

—Underline or circle key points.

—Make the font size easy to read—14 is best.

—Avoid the use of multiple fonts or multiple colors.

• Create a patient literacy panel that reviews the educational materials and processes used in the organization. (*See* Sidebar 9-5 on page 86.) Members of this panel can include nurses, patient safety professionals, and patients. At least one member of this panel should have low health literacy, so your organization can truly verify whether the materials you use are appropriate for the literacy level of patients. A litmus test for patient education material may involve asking an individual with low health literacy to edit new patient education materials by striking through every word he or she does not understand. If the individual can still understand the education material as edited, then the material is okay to use. If not, then more revision is necessary.

• Incorporate effective teaching methods for patients.

Sidebar 9-3. Plain Language

Professor Robert Eagleson defines *plain language* as a "clear, straightforward expression, using only as many words as are necessary. It is language that avoids obscurity, inflated vocabulary, and convoluted sentence construction. It is not baby talk, nor is it a simplified version of the English language. Writers of plain English let their audience concentrate on the message instead of being distracted by complicated language. They make sure that their audience understands the message easily."[13]

To clearly illustrate the concept of plain language look at the following two education pieces about the same program. One is written in plain language; the other is not.

Nonplain Language
The Acme Senior Day Program provides a safe and supportive environment where frail, dependent elders receive a program that is individually designed to reduce isolation and provides an alternative to premature institutionalization. If interested in taking advantage of this unique program, call 555-1111.
(This has a reading level of 17+.)

Plain Language
Could You Use Some Help?
Are You Lonely?
Does Your Health Make It Hard for You to Get Out?

The Acme Senior Day Program may be for you!
   Join us for fun activities planned just for you.
   Visit with other seniors.
   Have fun! We can pick you up.
   We serve lunch and snacks.
   Call us at 555-1111.
(This has a reading level equivalent to grade 6.)

Source: Audrey Riffenburgh, The Health Literacy Institute (http://www.healthliteracyinstitute.net/about.html). Used with permission.

This involves making education relevant and easy to understand and confirming patient understanding. As with written material, providers should use simple terms and short statements when speaking with patients and should avoid complicated medical jargon. Providers should slow down and give patients ample time to ask questions and express concerns. Other strategies include the following:

—Use the teach-back method to confirm patient understanding. This approach involves providers asking patients to state in their own words (teach back) key concepts, decisions, or instructions just discussed. If a patient

---

Sidebar 9-4. Informed Consent

Low health literacy can be particularly problematic when confronting the issue of informed consent. Recent studies about informed consent show that 60%–69% of patients do not read or understand the information contained in a hospital consent form. Even after giving consent, 18%–45% of patients are unable to recall major risks associated with a procedure, and 44% do not know the exact nature of their operation.[14] This creates a significant patient safety issue.

To prevent possible patient care issues, organizations should review their informed consent documents and ensure that they are written in an appropriate, easy-to-understand manner. If they are not, then revising the documents following the previously mentioned tips for improving written material (pages 83–84) is important.

It is important that these documents address patient needs as well as those of legal departments. Also, the revisions may actually improve the documents.

In addition, it may be helpful to test any new or revised documents with a sample of patients from diverse backgrounds. Some questions to ask within this test include the following:
- Given the time, were you able to finish reading the form?
- Can you describe what the form says? How easy is it for you to do that?
- Do you have any questions about the form? Was anything unclear?
- Were there any words on the form you did not understand?

Consider the following example. The first paragraph is an organization's original informed consent form. The second paragraph is the revision using shorter sentences and plain language.

Old
It has been explained to me that during the course of the operation, unforeseen conditions may be revealed that necessitate an extension of the original procedure(s) or different procedure(s) than those described above. I, therefore, authorize such surgical procedure(s) as are necessary and desirable in the exercise of the professional judgment. The authority granted under this shall extend to all conditions that do require treatment even if not known to Dr. _____ at the time the operation is commenced.

New
I understand the doctor may find other medical conditions he/she did not expect during my surgery or procedure. I agree that my doctor may do any extra treatments or procedures he/she thinks are needed for medical reasons during my surgery or procedure.

In addition to the consent form, your organization should review the process of educating patients about informed consent. Providers should use easy-to-understand language when explaining the procedure during the informed consent discussion and use the teach-back method to confirm understanding.

Source: Gail Nielsen, Iowa Health System. Used with permission.

---

can restate your instructions correctly, then the patient education you provided was effective. If not, then you need to explain the instructions again, using simple words and additional methods of education, such as pictures or brochures. The teach-back method can be repeated until you confirm the patient understands your message. If after two or three tries the patient still does not demonstrate understanding, then look for other explanations (beyond your teaching) about why the message is not understood. For patients who do not understand your message, the next step might be to give a referral to a patient educator, encourage the patient to bring a family member or friend to the next appointment, or make an appointment for a follow-up visit or phone call.[15]

You need to be very careful when using the teach-back method so that it is done in a non-shaming way. You need to frame it as a help to you and not imply that the patient didn't understand. For example, saying "I want to confirm that I've done a good job teaching" may be helpful. Another

approach may be to say, "I know your family is coming today. What do you plan to say to them about our session today?"

—Encourage patients to Ask Me 3™.[16] This program empowers patients to ask about three main concepts every time education is provided:

1. What's my main problem?
2. What should I do for that main problem?
3. Why is that important?

In addition to encouraging patients to ask these three questions, providers are encouraged to teach to these questions as well. For example, when teaching patients about falls and why it is important for them to call and ask for assistance when going to the bathroom, the provider should take the following approach:

1. What's my main problem? You at are at risk for falling, particularly on the way to the bathroom
2. What should I do for that main problem? When you

Sidebar 9-5. Iowa Health and the New Readers of Iowa

Several years ago, Iowa Health began to strategically focus on the issue of low health literacy. As part of this focus, the organization began networking with community groups about the issue. One such group was the New Readers of Iowa. This organization consisted of about 80 people who had been together for nearly 20 years working on issues related to literacy. The group had started as part of a grant program to bring together people who struggled with reading. It was a diverse group with varying educational levels and different reasons for low literacy, including dyslexia, English as a second language, and so forth.

Over time the group had started to take on projects, such as working with the state of Iowa to make the ballot easier to understand. Members of the group began to focus on the issue of health care. Iowa Health partnered with this group to improve patient education materials and the organization's approach to dealing with health literacy issues. One member, Archie Willard, became co-chair of Iowa Health's patient safety team and worked on projects such as reviewing written education materials, creating a mandatory learning module about health literacy, and improving the organization's wayfinding system.

Figure 9-1. Ask Me 3™

We Believe:
The more you know about your health, the better.

We Want You to Ask:
Your doctor, nurse, pharmacist or therapist questions about your health. Ask us to tell you in plain language:

❶ What is my main problem?
❷ What do I need to do?
❸ Why is it important for me to do this?

If You Don't Understand:
Tell us you don't understand.

We Want You to Understand.

For More Information on Clear Health Communication go to www.askme3.org.
Questions provided by the Partnership for Clear Health Communication.

Iowa Health uses this flier to help educate patients on the Ask Me 3 program.

Source: Iowa Health System. Used with permission.

need to go to the bathroom, call me using this call button here. Let me show you how to use it.

3. Why is it important? Because if you fall you could get hurt and we want to prevent you from getting hurt.

At the close of the teaching, providers should use the teach-back method to confirm that the patient understood what was taught. For example, you could say to the patient, "Your husband is coming to visit today, could you please tell me what you are going to tell him about the patient call button?" As the patient teaches back, the provider can identify gaps and teach to the gaps.

The Ask Me 3 program can not only help ensure patients receive the appropriate education, it can play an important role in creating a shame-free environment, as questions are welcomed and expected, and the program makes patients feel more comfortable and enhances communication with providers. (Figure 9-1, above, shows one organization's education tools for the Ask Me 3 approach.)

—Use return demonstration. "Return demonstration" or "show back" is another patient education method where the patient is asked to demonstrate to the caregiver how he

or she will do what was taught. This technique is used routinely in diabetic education and physical therapy.[17]

—Segment complex education. When patients require complex care and thus multifaceted education—such as with cardiac care or cancer treatment—you may want to break down education into manageable chunks and prioritize when specific information is taught. For example, in cardiac care, the first session may cover important medications and how patients can weigh themselves. After the patient is comfortable with this topic, a subsequent session may focus on diet and exercise. At the conclusion of each segment, providers should verify patient understanding and ask if the patient has any questions.

As you are designing and implementing revised patient education materials and teaching methods, establish performance measures to determine the success of these initiatives. Some of these measures may include the number of unplanned admissions, missed appointments, repeat visits, and medication errors.

Also give consideration as to how you educate and create awareness for patients and their families to be involved. Is it part of the admission process? How do you reinforce the message—posters, staff reminding patients, and so forth? Also, be aware that transitions of care, such as discharge, are critical times to engage patients and help ensure that they understand the process of their care. They are also great times to debrief the patient and their family to assess what their perception of the care experience is. Simple questions like, "What did we do well? What could we have done better? What would you like to see the next time?" fill two roles. They demonstrate that the organization cares, and they afford an opportunity to gather ideas for further improvement when they are fresh in the patient's mind.

REFERENCES

1. The Joint Commission: National Patient Safety Goal 2. http://www.jointcommission.org/PatientSafety/NationalPatientSafetyGoals (accessed Sep. 3, 2008).

2. The Joint Commission: National Patient Safety Goal 13. http://www.jointcommission.org/PatientSafety/NationalPatientSafetyGoals (accessed Oct.10, 2008).

3. Fahey L., Schilling L.: Nurse knowledge exchange: Patient hand-offs. *AAACN Viewpoint*, Sep.–Oct. 2007.

4. Joint Commission: Facts About Speak Up Initiatives. http://www.jointcommission.org/GeneralPublic/Speak+Up/about_speakup.htm (accessed Oct. 30, 2008).

5. Dana-Farber Cancer Institute: *Patient- and Family-Centered Care.* http://www.dana-farber.org/pat/pfac (accessed Oct. 1, 2008).

6. Institute for Family-Centered Care. http://www.familycenteredcare.org/about/inst.html (accessed Oct. 1, 2008).

7. U.S. Department of Health and Human Services, Office of Disease Prevention and Health Promotion: *Healthy People 2010.* http:// www.healthypeople.gov (accessed Oct. 10, 2008).

8. U.S. Department of Health and Human Services, Office of Disease Prevention and Health Promotion: *Quick Guide to Health Literacy.* http://www.health.gov/communication/literacy/quickguide/factsliteracy.htm (accessed Oct. 10, 2008).

9. Friedland R.: New estimates of the high costs of inadequate health literacy. In Proceedings of Pfizer Conference "Promoting Health Literacy: A Call to Action." Washington, D.C., Oct. 7–8, 1998.

10. Howard D.H., Gazmararian J., Parker R.M.: The impact of low health literacy on the medical costs of Medicare managed care enrollees. *Am J Med* 118:371–377, 2005.

11. Parikh N.S., et al.: Shame and health literacy: The unspoken connection. *Patient Educ Couns* 27:33–39, Jan. 1996.

12. Abrams M.A, et al.: *Reducing the Risk by Designing a Safer, Shame-Free Health Care Environment.* Chicago: American Medical Association, 2007.

13. Eagleson, R.: *Short Definition of Plain Language.* Plain Language Action and Information Network. http://www.plainlanguage.gov/whatisPL/definitions/eagleson.cfm (accessed Jul. 20, 2008).

14. Lorenzen B., Melby C., Earles B.: Using health literacy principles to improve the informed consent process. *AORN J* 88:23–29, 2008.

15. Osborne H.: Confirming understanding with teach-back technique. *Boston Globe.* http://www.boston.com/jobs/healthcare/oncall/articles/2007/11/20/confirming_understanding_with_the_teach_back_technique (accessed May 25, 2008).

16. National Patient Safety Foundation: *Ask Me 3.* http://www.npsf.org/askme3 (accessed Oct. 30, 2008).

17. Institute for Healthcare Improvement: *Transforming Care at the Bedside How-to Guide: Creating an Ideal Transition Home for Patients with Heart Failure.* http://www.ihi.org/IHI/Topics/MedicalSurgicalCare/MedicalSurgicalCareGeneral/Tools/TCABHowToGuideTransitionHomeforHF.htm (accessed Oct. 10, 2008).

Chapter Ten

USING TECHNOLOGY TO ENHANCE SAFETY

Karen Frush and *Asif Ahmad*

Technology is a double-edged sword. On one hand it can improve efficiency, enhance communication, improve documentation, and supplement a clinician's skills to provide truly exceptional care. On the other hand, if not used appropriately or if used in an environment that cannot support it, technology can lead to less efficiency, poor communication, decreased morale, safety risks, and ultimately patient error. Technologically spectacular systems can fail, and when they fail, they can fail spectacularly.

SAFETY COMES FIRST, TECHNOLOGY FOLLOWS

The key to using technology well is to have it enhance safety efforts; that is, safety efforts must drive the use of technology and not the other way around. In other words, technology must support your organization's safety goals not be the goal itself.

Technology works only if you have a culture based on teamwork and communication. Leaders and frontline staff must be able to work as a team to identify opportunities to use technology, as well as identify possible problems with the technology. Staff members must feel comfortable speaking up about potential problems and must believe that their opinions will be heard, respected, and responded to. Technology also requires a culture of learning in which front line providers and leaders alike are committed to continuous learning and improvement.

Successfully implementing technology, such as a computerized prescriber order entry system (CPOE) or bar-coding system, requires a systematic approach. (*See* Sidebar 10-1 for more information on the CPOE system.) Your organization should not rush through the process and should include multiple perspectives. Following are some

points to consider when systematically implementing technology:

• Don't just deploy technology and hope it improves outcomes. Instead you must critically examine the process or processes you hope to improve and do a total process reengineering. Within this reengineering, consider what is the most optimal way you need to function and then identify which technology you can use and adapt it for your culture. Creating a good process is the key. An ineffective process will still be ineffective even if it is automated. You should solve process problems first and then determine the appropriate technology that supports the solution.

• Sometimes technology is not the solution. In many cases—about 60% of the time—an organization's issues cannot be fixed through technology. When an organization faces underlying cultural issues, such as teamwork, accountability, or reliability problems, technology will not fix those issues and may, in fact, exacerbate them.

• Consider the process participants and gather feedback. To help in the reengineering process, your organization should consider creating a multidisciplinary team. Such a team allows multiple perspectives on an issue. As mentioned in Chapter 9, patients and their families may be critical members of these teams. For example, if your organization is working on processes to improve communication with patients, and you are considering implementing a patient portal, you should involve patients in the process redesign and technology implementation work. (*See* Sidebar 10-2 on page 91 for more information about a patient portal.)

Individuals who are most directly affected by a process should make up the brunt of any multidisciplinary team. Within these teams, your organization should also consider

---

Sidebar 10-1. Computerized Provider Order Entry

Some 40% of medication errors are caused by cognitive mistakes on the part of the prescribing physician, and illegible handwriting accounts for another 25%.[1] A computerized prescriber order entry system (CPOE) is a well-known computer-based technology that allows providers to enter medication orders, verify allergies, and identify drug interactions in order to improve efficiency and reduce error. When used effectively, a CPOE system can accomplish the following:

- Ensure that orders are legible and complete because they are entered into the computer and no longer written out by hand.
- Prevent prescribing errors, such as wrong dose, wrong drug, and wrong schedule of administration errors. CPOE programs often have forcing functions that help ensure that the correct dosage range is administered on the correct schedule.
- Identify allergies and drug interactions. CPOE systems can store allergy information and screen for adverse drug interactions.
- Bring evidence to the bedside. Those systems programmed with evidence-based care protocols and information can help physicians make care decisions easier and more accurately.

However, there are some potential downsides to these systems:

- Humans must calibrate the systems with allergy, drug interaction, and dosage information. If calibration is not accurate, you can systemically build errors into the medication process. Consider the computer that was programmed with the wrong standardized dose for treating infection in an infant. A baby was inadvertently given 500 times the recommended dose of antibiotic and died. Although the organization had a technically advanced system, it did not have the appropriate checks and balances and teamwork culture that would have allowed that system to operate effectively.
- CPOE limits teamwork. With such a system, a physician may sit in a room and complete his or her computer work. The need to speak and interact with the nurse and the pharmacist has decreased. For a CPOE system to work, organizations must examine how such a system will integrate into their current teamwork structure to ensure that valuable communication among nurses, physicians, pharmacists, and other team members is supported.
- CPOE implementation efforts often consider only how physicians will be impacted by the technology. When considering the workflow of a unit and how a CPOE system will affect the workflow, it is important to consider more than just physicians. While they are the predominant users of the system, the workflow of the nursing and pharmaceutical staff will also be affected by the system and thus should be considered.

---

involving information technology (IT) professionals. When working on improving a process or procedure, input on how technology could enhance that procedure can be very helpful. Including IT professionals on improvement teams can ensure that perspective is heard.

- Using an "off the shelf product" is not going to work. After you have revised and retooled a process and you determine that technology will supplement the solution, you must determine which technology to use. Every organization is different, and so the technology that works in one organization will most probably not work in another. Starting with an off-the shelf product is okay, so long as the IT department sees the technology as a starting point, not an end-all tool.

- The people using the tool must be involved in designing or customizing the tool. Not only does this ensure that the people using the tool get what they need out of the tool, but it makes a difference in frontline staff's ownership of and commitment to the technology. If staff members are not committed to the technology it can encourage workarounds, which can lead to unexpected errors and ultimately to patient harm.

- Not every technology is appropriate for every department. The intensive care unit (ICU) and the oncology department are alike in that they both provide care, treatment, and services to patients in a fast-paced and complex environment, and yet there are so many more differences than similarities. Taking a technology system that works in the ICU and applying it to oncology is an exercise in frustration and can lead to workarounds and patient error. When customizing technology, don't just figure out one approach for every unit, but map out the workflow of each unit that uses the technology and figure out how the technology can be adapted to fit that workflow.

- Spend time planning implementation. You should not underestimate the importance of effective implementation planning. Organizations should spend a fair amount of time on this process, to ensure smooth deployment. A helpful tool in this is a process map. Creating such a map allows you to outline the implementation strategy, including which units/areas will be implemented first, how you will measure success, what training needs will be necessary, and

---

Sidebar 10-2. Patient Portal

A patient portal is a relatively new technology, which allows patients to go online to a secure site and make appointments, pay their bills, check test results, view their medical record, request prescriptions, obtain referrals, and perform other personal health care tasks. Organizations can choose to create such a portal to help engage patients in their own care, improve communication with patients and their families, and help prevent errors associated with the failure to communicate about test results. Some organizations are hesitant to create such a system for fear it will intimidate patients. The fact is that if the information housed in such a system is important for the patient to know, then he or she should have access to it. This is not unlike financial management or travel management systems in which consumers can quickly access important personal information securely and quickly online.

When designing a patient portal system, organizations should consider their culture and whether such a system works within the culture and values of the organization. In addition, they should involve multiple perspectives in the design process, including physicians, nurses, patients, families, financial services, pharmacy, and so forth. The key to creating such a system? Determine and understand what patients really want out of the system, figure out how you can address those needs, and consider technology that helps with the solution.

---

how you will incorporate feedback into improvement. Organizations should not race through this planning process. By dedicating time to considering all the facets of implementation, you are more likely to have a smooth implementation.

- Deploy quickly. Although the planning process for purchasing, customizing, and implementing new technology will take time, the deployment process itself should be quick. This is, of course, dependent on effective prework. By having a speedy deployment you can maintain staff excitement and limit staff frustration.

- Technology implementation should not be a never-ending story. While implementation should occur in phases, you should move through those phases efficiently until the entire organization has the new technology. If you do partial implementation, you make the system more complicated and harder to handle.[2] If some functions are handled on paper while others are managed online, nurses and pharmacists will have to duplicate work as the project drags on, and excitement about the project will lag.

- Address glitches. Although your organization may have done extensive prework and workflow analysis, the likelihood that the technology will be a perfect fit when first deployed is slim. You should have systems in place to capture problems with technology, determine how to address those problems, and make alterations to address issues. Staff should be able to report problems through already existing reporting tools—executive walkarounds, a glitch book, and a safety-reporting system—but you also may want to have specific follow-up meetings or focus groups with staff to determine what needs fixing.

- Be creative. Fixing glitches often requires some creativity and out-of-the box thinking. *Consider this example: A large medical center was implementing a new CPOE system. After the system had "gone live," it was discovered that cardiologists who needed to admit a patient for cardiac catheterization could no longer write orders before the patient was formally admitted, because that was not allowed in the CPOE system. This caused patient delays and provider frustration. To address the problem, the implementation team created a "virtual unit" within the CPOE system that allowed the cardiologists to admit patients virtually. This technical solution was much easier than the political one of explaining to the admitting and billing offices why the cardiac unit needed to be able to "admit" patients on its own.*[2]

As previously mentioned, health care technology can help achieve fantastic outcomes; however, it can also be a contributing factor to error and harm. By keeping lines of communication open between leaders in technology—information systems professionals, biomedical engineers, and so forth—clinicians, and operational leaders, you can ensure that existing technology is functioning appropriately in a way that supports the safe delivery of care and that new technology acts as a supplement to safe and reliable care delivery.

REFERENCES

1. Lesar T.S., Briceland L., Stein D.S.: Factors related to errors in medication prescribing. *JAMA* 277:312–317, 1997.
2. Baker M.L.: Duke Health uses IT to get beyond doctors' handwriting. eWEEK, Mar. 23, 2005.

OTHER RESOURCES

1. Frush K.S.: Fundamentals of a patient safety program. *Pediatr Radiol.* 38(4):5633–5638, 2008.
2. Mekhjian H., et al.: Development of a web-based event reporting system in an academic environment. *J Am Med Inform Assoc.* 11(1):11–18, Jan.–Feb. 2004.

Chapter Eleven

AN EFFECTIVE STRATEGY FOR MEASUREMENT

Robert C. Lloyd

Measurement has become a central part of health care management and administration. This has not always been the case. The push for bringing measurement principles into the daily practice of health care professionals started in earnest in the early 1980s. This is when business groups, state and national agencies, and consumers began asking questions about health care outcomes, costs, and the patient experience.

To answer all of these questions, organizations required one crucial ingredient—data. According to Provost and Murray, "Data are documented observations or results of performing a measurement process. Data can be obtained by perception (for example, observation) or by performing a measurement process."[1]

THE CHANGING PERSPECTIVE ON PERFORMANCE MEASUREMENT

Over the past 25 years, measurement of health care processes and outcomes has been evolving and rapidly changing. Initially, the focus was primarily on collecting data and merely publishing summary statistics. Little was being done in the early and mid-1980s to make sense out of the data and produce information for decision making. Austin clarified this point by writing:

Data *refers to the raw facts and figures which are collected as part of the normal functioning of the hospital. Information, on the other hand, is defined as data, which have been processed and analyzed in a formal, intelligent way, so that the results are directly useful to those involved in the operation and management of the hospital.*[2]

Irrespective of how an individual interacts with the health care system, most would agree that it is information that is the desired end product, not just a table of raw data.

Whether you work at the bedside or in the lab, prepare medications in the pharmacy, perform surgery, make home care visits, or serve as the CEO of a large integrated delivery system, interpreting information has definitely become a central part of your daily work.

The Push for Transparency

The health care profession collects a lot of data. Some suggest that in our zeal to measure, monitor, and improve, we are drowning in data. But these data are typically collected at the patient level, during a patient visit, and measure the performance of the patient's body at a fixed point in time. The conclusions we can derive as a result of these individual measures are that at this fixed point in time, on this day, and at this hour, this is how this patient performed against selected benchmarks, such as blood pressure, cholesterol level, heart rate, or respiration rate.

This approach to measurement works well when we are asking questions about one patient; however, when the questions being asked are directed toward the health or well-being of a group of patients or the total population of a city, state, province, or country, then measurement moves to an entirely different level. Data collection methods and the way results are analyzed and displayed changes substantially.

As interest in health care measurement and data has moved from looking at individual data to asking questions about groups of patients, hospital- or clinicwide performance, or the health of a county, a new theme in measurement has emerged—transparency. As discussed in Chapter 1, transparency involves open and easy access to information; in this case, information about processes, outcomes, and providers. The assumption is that if patients and their families, as well as purchasers and insurers of health

Sidebar 11-1. Transparency Reveals Poor Performance

Prior to the recent push for transparency of health care data, data about outcomes were not collected or shared widely. Everyone merely assumed that health care in the United States was safe and reliable. Unfortunately, as more data have become available to the public and political leaders, the overall conclusion is that the U.S. health care system is not doing very well. For example, in the most recent Commonwealth Fund comparative report (*see* figure, below) the United States received an overall score of 66 out of a possible 100. If a child brought home a report card reflecting that score, most parents would be rather upset.

The inadequacies of the U.S. health system become even more obvious when the United States is compared to other nations. For example, when looking at the measure "mortality amenable to health care"— defined as "deaths before age 75 that are potentially preventable with timely and appropriate medical care"—the United States ranks 15th out of 19 countries. Contrast that with the amount of money the United States spends to achieve this dismal ranking, and these statistics are even more appalling.

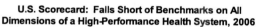

U.S. Scorecard: Falls Short of Benchmarks on All Dimensions of a High-Performance Health System, 2006

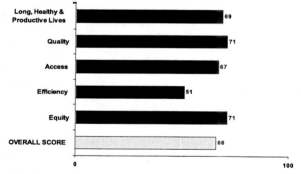

This figure illustrates the United States' poor performance in health care.

Source: Commonwealth Fund National Scorecard on U.S. Health System Performance, 2006. Used with permission.

care, are provided with full data on health care processes and outcomes, better decisions could be made. The argument has been that the health care community has not readily and openly shared performance data with those seeking health care services.

In today's era of ready Internet access and 24-hour media, consumers interested in purchasing a new car can get on the Internet and in 10 minutes find out all they need to know about the car they are thinking of buying. They can even get a rating of the "best" cars and see how the make and model they are considering compares to a larger class of similar cars. On the other hand, consumers needing to have their hip replaced have no clear way of determining which is the "best" hospital or group of surgeons to select for this procedure. The information is not only not readily available, it likely doesn't exist. Consequently, the need for transparency of health care information, such as outcomes, results, and even errors, has provided probably the largest single challenge in health care in recent time.

So the critical questions for your health care organization are these: Do you know your data and results better than anyone else? And do you have a way to turn that data into information and measure the quality of care you provide? If you do not, then it will be entirely too late to start thinking about your quality measurement journey when you are told there is a reporter from the local newspaper waiting in your office who wants to talk about your infection rates that have just been obtained from the state data commission. Do you have a road map to guide your quality measurement journey, or do you hope that the local reporters or TV crew pick the hospital down the street to interview? Hope is not a plan!

EMBARKING ON A QUALITY MEASUREMENT JOURNEY

Measuring quality is a journey, and like any journey there are various stops along the way. The following sections describe these stops. (Figures 11-1 and 11-2 on page 95 illustrate the concepts discussed below.) While the scope of this publication allows only a brief introduction to some of these stops, a list of references for further information can be found at the end of the chapter in Sidebar 11-2.

Setting Aims

First, to make data collection relevant, all measurement should be directly connected to your organization's mission or aim. You can test this yourself the next time you are working with an improvement team. Ask the members of the team if anyone can articulate which of the organization's aims are being maximized by the team's efforts? You will usually get blank stares when you ask this question. Some brave soul might respond, "I have no idea. We were told by

Figure 11-1. The Quality Measurement Journey

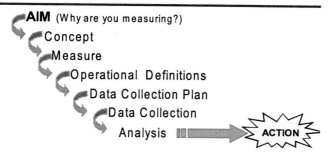

This figure illustrates the different stops along the quality measurement journey.

Source: R.C. Lloyd & Associates. Used with permission.

Figure 11-2. Examples of the Quality Measurement Journey

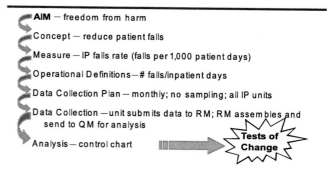

This figure provides examples for each stop along the journey.

Source: R.C. Lloyd & Associates. Used with permission.

our boss to improve this process." If the employees of an organization do not understand and appreciate how measurement connects their work to the organization's purpose and current strategic objectives, then they will be going through the motions but never connect the dots. Aims help answer the question, "Why are you measuring?"

Determining Concepts

An organizational aim may be to have freedom from harm. This is the type of statement you will find frequently in an organization's mission statement. From this aim emerge a variety of concepts that address different aspects of harm. Although concepts stem from high-level aims, they do not represent measurement. For example, the concept addressed in Figure 11-3 on page 99 is reducing patient falls. Although it is more specific than the aim, it is still not measurement. Reducing patient falls is a desired end state. It is not until you actually move to identifying a specific way to measure patient falls that you can actually take the first steps toward reducing them.

Selecting Measures

Within a concept, there are several potential measures that you can use to measure the concept. For example, if we stick with patient falls as the concept, we might consider the following measures:

• A count. You could merely count the number of falls in a defined period of time (for example, a day, a week, or a month). What does this give you? Is a count of the number

of falls the most appropriate way to measure the concept of a patient fall? This month your organization had 26 falls. Last month your organization had 37. What does this tell you? It becomes even more challenging when you compare two hospitals. Hospitals A and B each had 35 falls this month. Which one is better? You don't know because you have no context for the number of falls. If you are told, however, that Hospital A is a 530-bed urban teaching hospital and Hospital B is a 210-bed community hospital, you now have a context for the data and would most likely say that it is not quite fair to compare the two hospitals because of differences in bed size, volume, location, and so forth.

• A percentage. To compute the percentage of falls, you would need to define a denominator (for example, all inpatients that could possibly fall). The numerator would then be all the inpatients who fell during their hospitalization and then aggregated for a defined period of time, such as a month or six months. With these two numbers you could compute the percent of patients who fell during the last month. Because a patient could fall more than once during a hospitalization, however, the measure would not capture multiple falls.

A percentage is based on a binomial distribution. Measuring patient falls with a percentage, therefore, means that the team is not concerned with the specific number of times an individual patient fell but merely if the patient fell once or more. The question is simply, "Did this patient fall, yes or no?"

• A rate. This is the most frequently used measure to track the concept of patient falls. Like a percentage, a rate is still calculated by having a numerator and a denominator, but they are different from the ones defined for a percentage. A patient falls rate would have as the numerator all patient falls, including multiples, during a defined period of time, such as a month. The denominator would then be the total number of patient days in the month. This would produce an inpatient falls rate (for example, 3.2 falls per 100 patient-days).

Consider this example to help distinguish the differences between a percentage and a rate. A hospital with 210 discharges in a given month had a total of 47 of the 210 discharged patients fall once or more during their stay. From this information, you could conclude that 22.3% of the patients fell once or more (47 patient falls/210 patients = 22.3%). This is a straight percentage because you only know the percentage of patients who fell once or more, and multiple falls are ignored. Now, imagine that during the same month the actual total number of falls including multiples, was 65, and the number of patient days for the month equaled 5,621. When you divide the total number of falls by the total patient-days (65/5,621) you end up with .01156. Converting this ratio to a rate produces 11.56 falls per 100 patient-days. In this case, you have normalized the number of falls to a common denominator.

A percentage has the same type of unit in the numerator and denominator. In our previous example, the unit was patients. The question is, out of all patients how many of them fell? The distinguishing characteristic is whether they fell or not. In a rate calculation, you have two different types of units being compared. In our example, the two units were falls and patient-days. When you have two different types of units being used you cannot calculate a percentage.

Reaching Consensus on Operational Definitions

After we have selected the specific measures we want to apply to our improvement project, we then need to be very clear about the operational definition of each measure. According to Deming, "An operational definition puts communicable meaning to a concept. Adjectives like good, reliable, uniform, round, tired, safe, unsafe, unemployed have no communicable meaning until they are expressed in operational terms of sampling, test, and criterion. The concept of a definition is ineffable: It cannot be communi-

cated to someone else. An operational definition is one that reasonable men can agree on."[3]

Stated a little differently, an operational definition is a description, in quantifiable terms, of what to measure and the specific steps needed to measure it consistently. A good operational definition has the following characteristics:

• Gives communicable meaning to a concept or idea
• Is clear and unambiguous
• Specifies the measurement method, procedures, and equipment (when appropriate)
• Provides decision-making criteria when necessary
• Enables consistency in data collection

Again, using the concept of a patient fall, it is necessary to ask, "What is the operational definition of a fall?" All falls are not the same. There are partial falls, near falls, falls with injuries, falls without injuries, and assisted falls. What is the difference between a partial fall and an assisted fall? Do all providers agree on the characteristics of each one? If you sent out three people to collect data on partial falls would they all define a partial fall in the same way? Would the data be valid and reliable? Could you combine the data from the three people and have confidence that you were comparing apples to apples? If our operational definition of a partial fall met the five criteria listed above, our data would most likely be consistent from person to person. If the three people did not use consistent operational definitions, then you end up with fruit salad rather than apples compared to apples.

Developing a Data Collection Plan and Collecting Data

After reaching consensus on the operational definitions for your measures, the next steps in the quality measurement journey are to first develop a data collection plan and then go out and actually gather the data. These two steps frequently run into roadblocks because team members are not well versed in the methods and tools of data collection. An effective data collection plan should address the following questions[4]:

• What process(es) will be monitored?
• What specific measures will be collected?
• What are the operational definitions of the measures?
• Why are you collecting these data? What is the rationale for collecting these data rather than other types?
• Will the data add value to your quality improvement efforts?

- Have you discussed the effects of stratification on the measures? (*See* below for more information on stratification.)
- How often (frequency) and for how long (duration) will you collect the data?
- Will you use sampling? If so, what sampling design have you chosen? (More information on sampling can be found in the section beginning at the bottom of this page.)
- How will you collect the data? What methods will you use? Some possible methods include data sheets, surveys, focus group discussions, phone interviews, or some combination of these methods.
- Will you conduct a pilot study before you collect data for the entire organization?
- Who will collect the data? This is a critical question and unfortunately, most improvement teams ignore it.
- What costs (monetary and time costs) will be incurred by collecting these data?
- Will collecting these data have negative effects on patients or employees?
- Do your data collection efforts need to be taken to your organization's institutional review board for approval?
- What are the current baseline measures?
- Do you have targets and goals for the measures?
- How will the data be coded, edited, and verified?
- Will you tabulate and analyze these data by hand or by computer?
- Are there confidentiality issues related to the use of the results?
- How will these data be used to make a difference?
- What plan do you have for disseminating the results of your data collection efforts?

Before beginning to collect data, team members must have serious dialogue about these questions. In addition, team members must be familiar with and be able to use the following key skills:

- Stratification
- Sampling

Stratification

Stratification is the separation and classification of data into reasonably homogeneous categories. The objective of stratification is to create groupings that are as mutually exclusive as possible. Such groupings are intended to minimize variation between groups and maximize variation within a group of similar patients, procedures, or events. The objective of stratification is to drill down into the data to lend clarity to your analysis.

Stratification is also used to uncover patterns that may be suppressed when all of the data are aggregated. Stratification allows understanding of differences in the data that might be due to the following:

- Day of the week (Mondays are very different than Wednesdays.)
- Time of day (Turnaround time is longer between 9 A.M. and 10 A.M. than it is between 3 P.M. and 4 P.M.)
- Time of year (We treat more flu patients in January than June.)
- Shift (The process is different during the day shift than during the night shift.)
- Type of order (stat versus routine)
- Type of procedure (nuclear medicine films versus routine X-rays)
- Type of machine (ventilators versus lab equipment)

Stratification is more of a logical issue than a statistical issue. It requires talking with people who are familiar with the concept being measured, knowing how processes surrounding that concept work, and identifying where pockets of variation may exist.

If your organization is planning to collect data on the culture of patient safety, for example, you should consider stratification. At some point you will most likely want to see the aggregated results for the entire organization. But, as discussed in Chapter 2, the real value of improving the culture for patient safety comes with the ability to stratify the results by unit and employee categories, such as nurses, physicians, lab, pharmacy, or administration. It also might be very insightful to see if the culture scores differ by tenure within the organization, age of the employee, or the shift in which he or she works.

The critical point for successful stratification is that you think about the stratification levels or categories before you actually embark on gathering the data. After the data have been collected it is frequently too late or too time consuming to tease apart the stratification questions that may arise.

Sampling

Sampling—the second key skill needed during the data collection planning stage—involves collecting data on a portion of a total population and applying the data to the entire population.

Realize first of all that not every measure requires sampling. Sometimes there are small amounts of data, and sampling is not required or desirable. At other times you have ample data but the measure does not require that a subset of data be pulled from the total population. For example, if you want to know what percentage of patients receive appropriate medication reconciliation at the time of discharge, you would most likely take all the patients discharged during the week or month (the denominator) and ask, "How many of these patients received appropriate medication reconciliation?" (the numerator). When there is a fairly large amount of data, however, and you cannot afford to spend the time or money to capture every occurrence of data, then sampling is appropriate. The question is, how do you draw your samples?

All too often health care professionals are not well-versed in sampling methods. As a result, they end up collecting too much data, too little data, or data that do not reflect the population they are trying to measure.

There are two basic approaches to sampling: *probability* and *nonprobability*. While you can find very practical discussions of sampling methods in any basic text on statistical methods or research design, following is a brief description of the two approaches.

Probability Sampling

Probability sampling methods are based on a very simple principle: Within a known population of a specific size, there will be a fixed probability of selecting any single element in the population. The selection of this element (and subsequent elements) must be determined by objective statistical means if the process is to be truly random; in other words, not affected by judgment, purposeful intent, or convenience. There are four basic approaches to probability sampling:

• Systematic sampling. This type of sampling is achieved by numbering or ordering each element in the population—such as time order, alphabetical order, or medical record order—and then selecting every *k*th (k being a predetermined number) element. The key point that most people ignore when pulling a systematic sample is that the starting point for selecting every *k*th element should be generated through a random process. This approach has also been referred to as mechanical sampling.

• Simple random sampling. This is accomplished by giving every element in the population an equal and independent chance of being included in the sample. A random number generator or a random number table is usually used to devise a random selection process.

• Stratified random sampling. This results when stratification is applied to a population and then a random process is used to pull samples from within each strata. This approach helps to ensure that different groups within the population have a chance (probability) of being selected, which may not be the case with a simple random sample.

• Stratified proportional random sampling. This is a little more complex because it requires figuring out what proportion each stratum represents in the total population then replicating this proportion in the sample that is randomly pulled from each stratum. To successfully use this approach and stratified random sampling, you need to have sufficiently large populations so that you can divide them into smaller stratification levels and still have enough data from which to draw an appropriate sample. For example, if you stratify by gender, age, race, and prior hospitalization within the last 30 days, you may wind up with a category—such as black females over 65 that were in the hospital within the last 30 days—that contains only six patients. In this case, you have stratified by so many levels that you have reduced the number of patients to a point that sampling does not make sense.

Nonprobability Sampling Methods

Nonprobability sampling methods are usually used when the researcher is not interested in being able to generalize the findings to a larger population. The basic objective of nonprobability sampling is to select a sample that the researchers believe is "typical" of the larger population. A chief criticism of these approaches to sampling is that there is no way to factually measure how the nonprobability sample is representative of the population from which it is drawn. Samples pulled this way are assumed to be "good enough" for the people drawing the sample but the findings should not be generalized to larger populations.

• Convenience sampling is the classic "man on the street" interview approach to sampling. In this case, a reporter may select four or five people standing on the train platform (who look interesting or approachable) and ask them what they think of the local school referendum. While

Figure 11-3. The Process of Turning Data into Information for Decision Making

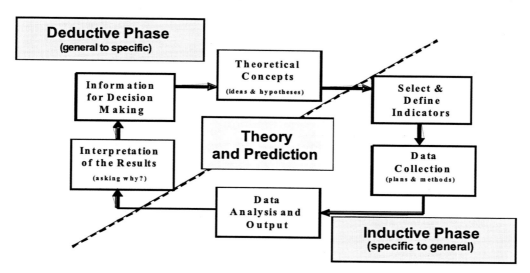

This figure illustrates how your organization can move from data to information for decision making.

Source: Adapted from Lloyd, R.: *Quality Health Care: A Guide to Developing and Using Indicators.* Boston: Jones & Bartlett Publishers, 2004. Used with permission.

these interviews may provide interesting sound bites, they should not be used to arrive at a conclusion that "this is how the people feel on this issue."

• Quota sampling is frequently used with convenience sampling. When this is done the reporter referenced above knows that he or she needs to get a total of 4 sound bites (the quota) that the producer can use. So he or she is focused on getting these 4 interviews; not 3 and not 5 but a quota of 4. This type of sampling is done frequently in health care settings, such as when a quota of 10 charts or 8 patient interviews is set as the desired amount of data. There are steps that can be taken in developing quota samples to ensure reasonably robust data.[5] Unfortunately, most of the time these steps are not followed, and quota sampling represents a fairly weak approach to sampling.

• Judgment sampling is frequently used in quality improvement initiatives. Judgment sampling relies on the knowledge of subject matter experts. These individuals can tell you when the performance of a process varies and when this variation should be observed. For example, if the admitting clerk tells you that patients "bunch up" between 0830 and 0930 and that this is a very different situation than what she observes between 1500 and 1600, then you should con-

sider sampling differently during these two time periods. Similarly, if a staff nurse tells you that "things get crazy around here at 1100 due to discharge timing" then you would want to create a sampling plan for "crazy time" and "non-crazy time." The critical point for judgment sampling is that the person offering the judgment needs to be credible and respected by those working in the process. Otherwise, bias increases dramatically in this form of sampling.

Building knowledge of sampling methods is one of the best things you can do to enhance your data collection plan and processes. Good sampling techniques help to ensure the validity and reliability of the data you will take to the next step in your quality improvement journey—analysis.

Analyzing Data

Analyzing data is a critical process in the journey of quality measurement. (*See* Figure 11-3, above.) Within this process, data must be interpreted and placed in the appropriate context, otherwise it is an exercise with no real purpose. Remember that data collection and statistical analysis of the data are not the objectives in the quality measurement process. Data and its analysis provide a springboard for the real objectives—learning and improvement.

Unfortunately, many performance improvement teams fail to plan for and engage in the data analysis and interpretation stages of the quality measurement journey. Such planning and engagement requires thinking about the following questions:

- Who will be responsible for organizing the data after it is collected?
- If the data have been manually collected who will be responsible for assembling all the data collection forms?
- Did you remember to place a unique identification number on each chart, survey, or log sheet?
- If appropriate, have you set up a codebook for the data?
- How will you enter the data into the computer? Will you scan the data into a computer, enter it manually, or create an automatic download from an existing database?
- Who will enter the data? Will you verify the data after they have been entered? If you have a large volume of data—like the volume generated by surveys—have you considered using a professional data entry service?
- Who will be responsible for analyzing the data? (This question applies whether you are performing manual or automated analysis.)
- What computer software will you use? Will you produce descriptive statistical summaries, cross-tabulations, graphic summaries, or control charts?
- Do you have control charting software?
- After you have analyzed the data, who will be responsible for translating the raw numbers into information for decision making?
- Will you need to develop a written summary of the results? If so, who will be given this responsibility?
- Are there different audiences that need to receive the results, and have they requested different report formats?

Probably the biggest challenge your quality improvement team will face at this step is whether you will approach the analysis of data from a static or dynamic point of view. Most health care professionals have received statistical training that is grounded in static approaches to data. Static approaches to data analysis are designed to compare the results from the first time period (for example, the medication error rate last month) with the results at the second time period (this month) and raise the question "Are the two numbers different?" Research conducted in this manner is referred to as *static group comparisons*.[6] It is a pretty well-established fact that if you compare two numbers, there is a fairly high likelihood that one number will be different from the other. Some analysts and managers will apply the "interocular test of significance" and conclude that the two numbers certainly look different. If you want to be a little more precise, however, you will apply statistical tests of significance to see if the two data points are statistically significant at the .01 or .05 level of significance.

Static group comparisons, while quite popular in health care, are not the preferred approach when conducting quality improvement research. The best analytic path to follow for quality and safety is one guided by statistical process control methods (SPC). Statistical analysis conducted with SPC methods looks at variation in a process or outcome measure over time, not at fixed points in time. This branch of statistics was developed by Dr. Walter Shewhart in the early 1920s while he worked at Western Electric Company.[7] Shewhart's primary analytic tool, the control chart, serves as the cornerstone for all quality improvement work.

Because variation exists in all processes (consider your morning commute time, for example), the use of Shewhart control charts allows the researcher to analyze the data as a continuous stream that has a rhythm and pattern. Statistical tests are used to detect whether the process performance reflects what Shewhart classified as *common cause variation* or *special cause variation*. Decisions about improvement strategies and their impacts will be based on understanding the type of variation that lives in the process, not on whether one data point is different from another.

Shewhart control charts, therefore, are more like electrocardiogram readouts or patterns of vital signs seen on telemetry monitors in intensive care units. They are plots of data arranged in chronological order. The mean or average is plotted through the center of the data, and then the upper control limit and lower control limit (basically plus and minus three standard deviations around the mean) are calculated from the inherent variation that lives in the data. The control limits are not set by the individual constructing the chart. If appropriate, the variation in the chart can be compared to targets or other comparative reference data.

TAKING ACTION

The final step in the quality measurement journey involves taking *action* to make improvements. All the preceding steps are designed to lead to this outcome. Data without a context

---

Sidebar 11-2. References for Further Information

Following is a list of sources for more information on measurement, including information about measurement tools, statistical analysis methods, the statistics associated with health care performance in the United States, and so forth.

Austin C.: *Information Systems for Hospital Administration,* Chicago: Health Administration Press, 1983.

Babbie E.R.: *The Practice of Social Research,* Belmont, CA: Wadsworth, 1979, p. 196.

Benneyan J., Lloyd R., Plsek P.: "Statistical Process Control as a Tool for Research and Health Care Improvement." *Journal of Quality and Safety in Health Care* 12(6):458–464, 2003.

Carey R.: *Improving Healthcare with Control Charts,* Milwaukee: ASQ Quality Press, 2003.

Carey R., Lloyd R.: *Measuring Quality Improvement in Healthcare: A Guide to Statistical Process Control Applications,* Milwaukee: ASQ Quality Press, 2001.

Deming W. E.: *Out of the Crisis,* Cambridge, MA: MIT Press. 1992. pp. 276–277.

Lloyd R.: *Quality Health Care: A Guide to Developing and Using Measures,* Sudbury, MA: Jones and Bartlett, 2004.

Lloyd R.: "The Search for a Few Good Indicators," chapter 5 in *The Healthcare Quality Book: Vision, Strategy and Tools.* Edited by Ransom, S., Joshi M., Nash, D., Chicago: Health Administration Press, 2005. p. 101.

Mohamed M.A., Worthington P., Woodall W.H.: "Plotting Basic Control Charts: Tutorial Notes for Healthcare Practitioners" *Journal of Quality and Safety in Health Care.* 17:137–145, April 2008.

Provost L., Murray S.: *The Data Guide,* Austin, TX: Associates in Process Improvement and Corporate Transformation Concepts, 2007.

Schoen C., Davis K., How S.K.H, Schoenbaum S.C.: "U.S. Health System Performance: A National Scorecard" *Health Affairs.* 25(6):457–475, 2006.

Schultz L.: *Profiles in Quality,* New York: Quality Resources, 1994.

Western Electric Co.: *Statistical Quality Control Handbook,* Indianapolis: AT&T Technologies, 1985.

Wheeler, D.: *Advanced Topics in Statistical Process Control,* Knoxville, TN: SPC Press, 1995.

Wheeler D., Chambers D.: *Understanding Statistical Process Control,* Knoxville, TN: SPC Press, 1992.

---

or plan for action give the team a false sense of accomplishment. It is not until you identify change concepts that you believe will improve performance, and conduct tests of change, that the journey is complete. All too often health care managers and leaders see data as the beginning and end of the journey. The data merely allow us to set the direction of our improvement journey, not define where the journey will take us.

REFERENCES

1. Provost L., Murray S.: *The Data Guide,* Austin, TX: Associates in Process Improvement and Corporate Transformation Concepts, 2007.
2. Austin C.: *Information Systems for Hospital Administration,* Chicago: Health Administration Press, 1983.
3. Deming W.E.: *Out of the Crisis,* Cambridge, MA: MIT Press. 1992, pp. 276–277.
4. Lloyd R.: "The Search for a Few Good Indicators" In Ransom S., Joshi M., Nash D. (eds.): *The Healthcare Quality Book: Vision, Strategy and Tools.* Chicago: Health Administration Press, 2005.
5. Babbie E.R.: *The Practice of Social Research,* Belmont, CA: Wadsworth, 1979, p. 196.
6. Benneyan J., Lloyd R., Plsek P.: Statistical process control as a tool for research and health care improvement *Journal of Quality and Safety in Health Care* 12:458–464, 2003.
7. Schultz L.: *Profiles in Quality,* New York: Quality Resources, 1994.

Chapter Twelve

CARE PROCESS IMPROVEMENT

Terri Simmonds, Carol Haraden, **and** *David Munch*

Standardizing procedures, introducing structured communication techniques, implementing Executive WalkRounds™, redesigning patient education materials, deploying a computerized prescriber order entry system. What do all these actions have in common? They all involve improvement. Taking what was and making it better. Putting in the new to replace or enhance the old. While it is easy to say we must improve our processes, without a systematic approach to doing that, such efforts can and probably will fail. At the very least they will not go as smoothly as they should, and the resulting processes will not be as good as they could be.

There are many different ways to structure the improvement process; far too many, in fact, to be covered completely by this book. However, the following sections will look at some common methods that have been used successfully across many types of health care organizations within many different types of processes.

THE MODEL FOR IMPROVEMENT

Developed by Associates in Process Improvement and recommended by the Institute for Healthcare Improvement, the Model for Improvement is a straightforward effective tool for accelerating change.[1] The model has two main parts:

1. The following three fundamental questions, which organizations must address for each process being improved:
   a. What are we trying to accomplish?
   b. How will we know that change is an improvement?
   c. What changes can we make that will result in improvement?

2. The Plan-Do-Study-Act (PDSA) cycle to test and implement changes: The PDSA cycle guides the change process and helps determine if a change results in an improvement.

To answer the previous questions and drive improvement forward, you must engage in the following activities:

- Establish a team. Including the right people on a process improvement team is critical to a successful effort. Although teams can vary in size and composition, they should include individuals familiar with all the different parts of the process to be improved, including physicians, pharmacists, nurses, and other frontline workers, as well as managers and administrators. The team must include individuals representing three different kinds of expertise within your organization: system leadership, technical expertise, and day-to-day leadership. Without these different kinds of input, improvement will not move forward effectively.

A system leader has enough authority in your organization to institute a change that has been suggested and overcome barriers that arise. He or she has the authority to allocate the time and resources for the project and understands both the implications of a proposed change for various parts of the system and the more remote consequences that a change might trigger.

A clinical technical expert is someone who knows the subject being addressed intimately and understands the processes of care associated with that subject. An expert on improvement methods can provide additional technical support to a performance improvement team by helping the team determine what to measure, assisting in design of simple, effective measurement tools, and providing guidance on collection, interpretation, and display of data.

A day-to-day leader is the driver of the project, assuring that tests are implemented and overseeing data collection. It is important that this person understands not only the details of the system under study, but also the various effects of making change(s) in the system.

• Clearly state the goals or aims of the performance improvement project. A project aim should be specific, numerical, and measurable. It should describe the system to be improved and the patient population affected by the improvement, and it should be tied into the organization's strategic goals and values. It should set a time line for achievement and communicate that maintaining the status quo is not an option. Setting such aims helps to create tension for change, directs measurement, and focuses initial changes. An example of a well-defined aim might be to "reduce adverse events in the intensive care unit (ICU) by 75% within 11 months" or "achieve 100% compliance with the Universal Protocol within the next six months." Team members must agree on the aims of a project and be careful not to deliberately back away or "drift" away from an aim unconsciously. Regular repetition of the aim can help prevent this.

• Establish measures. As discussed in Chapter 11, by developing specific measures, creating a data collection plan, and collecting data to measure the success in meeting identified aims, organizations can determine whether an initiative actually leads to an improvement.

• Identify changes that are most likely to result in improvement. While not all changes lead to improvement, all improvement requires change. Changes that work in your environment will most likely stem from some general approaches or concepts that have worked in other organizations. While there are literally hundreds of change concepts from which you can develop specific changes, following is a brief list of some of the more common concepts:

— Eliminate waste. This involves systematically looking for ways of eliminating any activity or resource in your organization that does not add value. A critical tool in eliminating waste is Lean Methodology. (*See* a further discussion of Lean Methodology on pages 106–110.)

— Improve workflow

— Optimize inventory. This ties in neatly with reducing waste, as inventory of all types is a possible source of waste in organizations.

— Change the work environment. This could include both the physical environment and the cultural environment.

— Improve your relationship with patients.

— Manage time. This may include wait times, turnover times, or lead times. For example, organizations may focus on changes that decrease delays in the emergency department (ED) waiting room, improve the turnover times of operating rooms, or decrease the lead times necessary for critical tests.

— Reduce variation. As discussed in Chapter 4, reducing variation—also known as standardization—improves the predictability of outcomes and helps reduce the frequency of poor results.

— Increase reliability. Organizations can reduce errors by redesigning processes to make it less likely for people to make errors. This may involve implementing checklists, closed-loop communication cycles, or other such tools.

• Test changes on a small scale. After generating change ideas, test a change or group of changes on a small scale to see if they result in improvement. *Small scale* means such tests may involve 1 individual or 10 individuals, but invariably involve a smaller number than suggested by clinicians with limited improvement expertise. Small tests of change are never successes or failures, they are simply an opportunity for learning. There are many reasons to test changes, including the following:

— Tests verify that a change will result in improvement.

— Tests predict how much improvement can be expected from a change.

— Tests identify areas for improvement that can be quickly addressed on a more reasonable scale.

— Tests can help minimize resistance upon full implementation.

When beginning to test changes, you should pick easy changes to try. Look for the concepts that seem most feasible and will have the greatest impact.

Teams should test changes using the the Plan-Do-Study-Act model. This model was first developed by Walter A. Shewhart as the Plan-Do-Check-Act (PDCA) cycle. W. Edwards Deming modified Shewhart's cycle to PDSA, replacing "Check" with "Study." Within the model there are four main steps.

— Step 1: Plan. This step involves planning for the test of change. Within this step teams should answer the following questions:

○ What is the objective of the test?

○ What do we predict will happen during the test and why?

○ How will we perform the test?

○ Who will be involved? It's best to start the first PDSA cycle with willing participants. Some individuals are more enthusiastic to work with new ideas than others. According to Evert Rogers, these individuals are called early adopters and innovators, and they enjoy the experience of tweaking a process or idea until it works in their environment. On the flip side, late adopters are individuals who throw up roadblocks or downright refuse to try a new process or approach unless they are certain that all the potential pitfalls, complications, and problems with the process have been addressed.[2] When testing a change, you should work with the early adopters first and then work through the rest of the population, ultimately introducing the process to the late adopters.

○ When will we perform the test?

○ Where will we perform the test?

○ How will we measure success? What measures will we use and how will we collect data?

—Step 2: Do. This step involves carrying out the test on a small scale. During the "Do" step, team members should document problems and unexpected observations and begin to analyze the data

—Step 3: Study. As discussed in Chapter 11, data analysis is critical to any improvement project. Team members should set aside time to review data, see how they compare to the predictions, and summarize what was learned. Teams should reflect on the results of every change. After making a change, a team should ask: What did we expect to happen? What did happen? Were there unintended consequences? What was the best thing about this change? The worst? What might we do next? Too often, people avoid reflecting on failure. Remember that teams often learn very important lessons from tests of change that don't achieve what is predicted.

—Step 4: Act. Based on the results of the previous step, the Act step involves refining the change and preparing for the next test. If the test shows that a change is not leading to improvement, that knowledge is important too. "Failed" tests of change are a natural part of the improvement process; they indicate a direction to not go. If a team experiences very few failed tests of change, it is probably not pushing the boundaries of innovation very far.

Small tests of change are just that—small. It is better to conduct more PDSA cycles of small changes than fewer cycles of bigger changes. *Consider the following example of how one team used PDSA to test a small change. A 250-bed community hospital was working on a program to implement planned patient visits for blood sugar management. To test the change on a small scale, the organization worked with a physician who was excited about the program and willing to participate in the change process. She implemented the following PDSA test:*

Plan: Ask one patient if he or she would like more information on how to manage his or her blood sugar.

Do: Dr. J. asked her first patient with diabetes on Tuesday.

Study: Patient was interested; Dr. J. was pleased at the positive response.

Act: Dr. J. will continue with the next five patients and set up a planned visit for those who say "yes."

The tempo with which the repeating tests of change occurs will determine the speed with which the actual process becomes more reliable. Testing every day or every other day results in a key process improvement every couple of weeks. Testing once a week results in key process improvement every three to four months. The speed of testing is the key to speed of implementation and spread.

• Implement changes. After testing a change on a small scale, learning from each test, and refining the change through several PDSA cycles, the team can implement the change on a broader scale—for example, for an entire pilot population or on an entire unit. During implementation, teams learn valuable lessons necessary for successful spread, including key infrastructure issues, optimal sequencing of tasks, and working with people to help them adopt and adapt to a change.

• Spread the changes. After successful implementation of a change for a pilot population or an entire unit, the team can spread the changes to other parts of the organization or in other organizations. For example, if all 30 nurses on a pilot unit successfully implement a new medication reconciliation and order form, then spread would be replicating this change sequentially in all nursing units in the organization and assisting the units in adopting or adapting the change.

By using the Model for Improvement to drive improvement, organizations can quickly implement changes that achieve measurable results. As long as team members have change ideas to try, this model is effective at testing and implementing to achieve success.

LEAN METHODOLOGY

Toyota Production System or "Lean" production is an effective method for advancing patient safety by process design that achieves reliability through standard work, mitigation, and continuous improvement. Typically, Lean focuses on speed, elimination of waste, standardization, and flexibility/responsiveness.

Lean is not just a tool for process improvement, but is an organizational approach to reliability based on a set of explicit guiding principles that guide workers to provide defect-free workmanship.[3] It is also about tapping into the wisdom and motivation of the frontline worker to continually learn and improve based upon providing value to the customer with the least amount of waste possible. Although often used to improve clinical processes and systems, this philosophy and tools are equally applicable in "soft process" areas, such as new product development, employee orientation, accounting/finance, and customer service.

When improving a process using Lean Methodology, your organization must first start with a high-level analysis of the particular service line being examined from a customer value perspective. (*See* Sidebar 12-1 for some examples of processes that were improved using Lean.) The patient's journey through the clinical process is mapped step by step from beginning to end. This sequence of process steps, which are intended to provide value to the patient, is called the Value Stream and is recorded in the Value Stream Map. The map is then analyzed and the sequence of processes is segregated into process groups or "chunks" that can now be improved through a series of "Rapid Improvement Events" (RIEs).

Rapid Improvement Event

A Rapid Improvement Event is a two- to four-day event in which a process or a component of a process is analyzed and improved through the work of an integrated team. The RIE serves several purposes:

1. To improve and standardize a particular process, reduce waste, and improve reliability using Lean principles

---

Sidebar 12-1. Examples of Lean Improved Processes

Example: Our pharmacy evaluated the medication ordering process and found 142 steps in the current state. The future state had only 100 steps arranged in a much more efficient order and less chance of error.

Example: Pharmacists were spending an inordinate amount of time searching for lab values in the lab data system for their assessments of medication orders. The computers were programmed to automatically bring the information to the screen, doubling the efficiency of the pharmacist in the order review process.

Example: Shift change between nurses was observed. The receiving nurse was relying upon the verbal report and the patient information found in the electronic record. The off-shift written nursing summary was not being used because it was redundant, yet had been "tradition." This portion of the handoff process was stopped altogether, saving significant time in duplicate documentation.

Example: Chemotherapy infusion orders were evaluated for adjustments for weight and kidney function, and gaps were observed. Protocols and forcing functions were implemented to assure first-time quality.

---

2. To grow the team's knowledge of Lean methods and problem-solving skills through just-in-time training and the experience of the RIE.

3. Over the course of time, with multiple RIEs involving multiple members of the service line, cultural change takes place. Adherence to standard work and the skills for improvement become values and practices that are strengthened over time. A learning organization evolves.

Steps Involved with a Rapid Improvement Event

There are several steps involved in a RIE. Different organizations can take various approaches to these steps. The following sections take a brief look at one way to approach the steps.

Preparation: Preparation for RIEs starts with a planning phase in which leaders select improvement team members and prepare the team members for the event. Team members establish baseline measures, solicit input from members of the service line, schedule the improvement event, and determine implementation time lines.

The majority of the RIE team members come from the front line because they are the people who do the work.

They have the most in-depth understanding of the current work and the most knowledge of the opportunities for improvement. Their contribution on the team provides for greater improvement and comes with credibility that cannot be achieved with a top down approach. Because of their participation, it is much more likely that sustained improvement will be realized. Each RIE team has a lead, a facilitator, and an executive champion assigned to support the work. The lead's major responsibility is to manage the project to completion. The facilitator is skilled in facilitation methods and serves to guide the process of the RIE and ensure that all members participate. The executive champion participates on the team and supports the team's work, addressing barriers if they occur.

Step 1: The current state analysis is performed. At the beginning of the RIE, the agenda for the event is reviewed, team-building exercises take place, and norms are established. This is followed with just-in-time teaching for the improvement team for approximately one hour with a review of Lean principles and tools. The RIE that follows imbeds these skills into the team members thus providing experiential training.

When these activities are completed, the "current state" is analyzed. This is done by first writing each step in a particular process on a sticky note and placing it on the wall. Each step is placed in order, and if there is variability of a particular step, the variations are stacked vertically on the first variation. Rework loops are drawn and the layout of the floor, movement patterns, material locations, and work patterns are evaluated. The process is evaluated for evidence of waste using the following categories:

- Over-processing
- Waiting
- Excess inventory
- Excess movement of people
- Excess transport of materials
- Defects
- Overproduction of services or product
- Unused employee creativity

The learning proceeds and awareness grows. At the start, members of the team rarely have the same perception of the current process. The sharing of perceptions forces the realization of the previously unappreciated variability and brings the team to a common mental model of the current state.

In addition, this mapping process is not complete until the improvement team goes to where the work is performed and observes the process directly to see if the map they created in the classroom is an accurate representation of the work. It never is. Invariably, additions and revisions occur based upon direct observation. Observing the process helps the team visually appreciate the profound variability and unnecessary complexity of the process in which they work. The waste becomes apparent.

Process and outcome measures of the current state are determined, and data are collected either before or during this step. Future measures are determined to track the effectiveness of the new process, the implementation plan, and the evidence that improvement is being sustained.

Step 2: The future state is developed. After they analyze the current state of the process and agree upon a common mental model, the team evaluates each step in the process using the following criteria:

1. Does this step bring value to the customer?: "Value Add" ←→ "Non Value Add (NVA)"

2. If not, is it necessary?: "Non Value Necessary" ←→ Non Value Unnecessary"

The ratio of value added to NVA steps is typically 1 to 10, a remarkably low number.

After evaluating all the steps, the team then proceeds to take away the NVA unnecessary steps, occasionally taking out whole groups of steps that can be done in a more efficient manner. Team members evaluate and redesign remaining processes, taking out waste using Lean principles to provide more effective work. Some of the more common Lean principles used in the redesigning include:

- Base management decisions on long-term philosophy and core values, even at the expense of short-term financial goals. (Principle 1)

- Create process "flow" to surface problems. Design the sequence of services to be given one at a time in a smooth order. Waiting between steps or defects of steps will be more easily identified. (Principle 2)

- Use pull systems to avoid overproduction. Design the process to provide the service only when needed. (Principle 3)

- Level out the workload (*Heijunka*). Variable workload overwhelms the staff and increases the likelihood of error. Design processes to match capacity with demand and level demand as much as possible. (Principle 4)

- Stop when there is a quality problem (*Jidoka*).

Design systems to recognize defect or error immediately and respond immediately. (Principle 5)

• Standardize tasks for continuous improvement. This is a cornerstone of many organizations' design efforts and allows them to have predictability and reliability of work. It also allows for effective evaluation of a process when considering a design improvement. (Principle 6)

• Use visual control so no problems are hidden. Make the process as visible as possible so you can effectively identify process problems or compliance variance. (Principle 7)

• Use only reliable, thoroughly tested technology. As discussed in Chapter 10, it is important to address process problems first and not assume that a technology will fix a broken process. If you are introducing a new technology, use Lean to ensure that it is implemented into the work processes effectively.

Teams hold "stakeholder" sessions at the end of steps 1 and 2 where the improvement team's colleagues from the service line get to review the work and provide input. This is a critical step to build ownership and buy-in for the larger clinical team.

Step 3: The test of change is performed and observed. After a process has been redesigned, the new process is tried on the unit under direct observation of the team members. Members from the unit get to participate in this test and provide input. The information and measures from this test are evaluated and are used to improve the future state of the process design.

Step 4: The new process is finalized, including implementation plan, metrics, time lines, and roles. The project plan is set in this step starting with the implementation and communication plans. The team makes plans to observe the implementation on a regular basis, such as daily, weekly, monthly, and then quarterly. Assignments are made, resources are aligned. Support departments are commonly brought in at this time. For example, the facilities team may need to move a piece of equipment, information technology may need to add a computer terminal, and data support may need to develop a report.

Step 5: The communication plan to stakeholders is developed. A "Celebration" is held where the executive team, directors, members from the involved service line, and other interested parties come to hear about the RIE activity, the new process that has been developed, the improvements expected, and the plans for implementation. Learning

occurs here. Directors and others have the opportunity to evaluate the ideas for their areas, to understand their role in supporting this work, and to see that the organization is serious about improvement. This is one of the first opportunities for acknowledgment and validation in a meaningful way. Within this step, questions are asked and understanding grows. One of the more common questions asked of the team is: "What have you learned?"

Step 6: The new process is implemented. During this step, the team manages organizationwide implementation. Management plays a critical role in this phase and must be knowledgeable of the new work and able to coach the staff. Project management skills are critical here, and leadership support will be needed if the team is early in its Lean journey. The new standard process is observed daily for 2 to 4 weeks. If process control is achieved, the observations become less frequent over the course of 3 to 12 months. Coaching the staff to the new standard process occurs within this step.

The team must also be able to revise the standard process if an unanticipated issue surfaces that justifies a revision. It is critical here to improve and adhere to a standard process and not reach for a workaround.

It is also important to make the work as visible as possible, tracking the measures such that everyone can see them. Visual control boards and data walls are effective for making work visible. It is important to keep data simple and understandable. It may be helpful to use tally sheets, run charts, bar graphs, colors, and any method that identifies defects quickly such that response can be immediate.

Step 7: The plan for sustaining the work is developed. This is a critical phase requiring ongoing support and vigilance. There are many variables that determine sustainable success, including the strength of organization leadership, management, staff, organizational goals, clarity/alignment to the standard work, information management, and others. Some process designs will require more work than others. For example, if the work has forcing functions, there will be less need for vigilance because choice and opportunity to deviate from the standard are restricted.

Improvements that are not sustained are an enormous drain on human resources. All previous efforts that have gone into improving the process are wasted, and the culture of workarounds is reinforced. Consequently, planning for an improvement event requires a plan to sustain the work.

Figure 12-1. An Example of the A-3 Tool

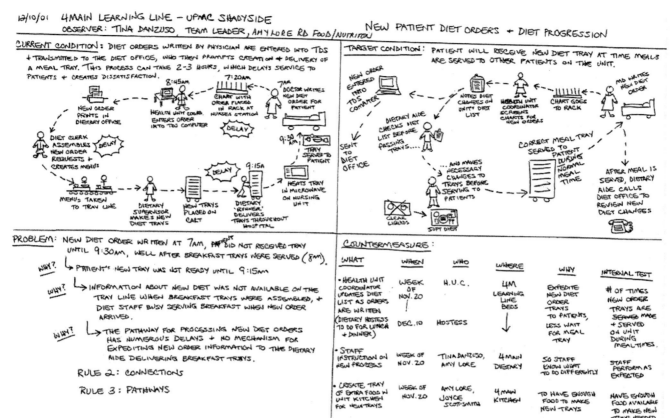

This figure shows one organization's A3 approach to analyzing and addressing issues surrounding new patient diet orders.

Source: Tami Merryman, UPMC Shadyside, Pittsburgh, PA. Used with permission.

Solving Problems on a Daily Basis

In addition to using RIEs, Lean can be used for small-scope problem solving on a day-to-day basis via the "A3" tool. (*See* Figure 12-1, above.) This method uses an 11 by 17 piece of paper divided in half. On the left side of the paper you state the problem, draw the current state using pictures, determine the root causes of the problem, and list the types of process waste observed. The right side of the paper is for recording the owner and coach to solve the problem, the solution(s) developed (again using pictures if possible), implementation plan, communication plan, measures, and time lines. Critical to the A3 process are conversations among the stake holders that build consensus by contributing to the analysis and coming to agreement on the solution. When agreement is achieved, the problem can be solved.

Within both the larger-scale RIE and the smaller-scale A3, similar steps are used. These approaches force a deeper thought process to occur in the analysis of a problem and the determination of a solution, thereby achieving better solutions and reducing waste. Both approaches build in project management discipline for successful implementation, and both approaches create learning.

Lean Methodology Advances an Organization Toward High Reliability

Through a foundation of standard work, visual management, and leveled production, Lean allows processes to be developed that are reliable, safe, and supportive of people in the health care environment. Waste is reduced, quality is built into the workflow and efficiencies follow. Those hospitals that provide the leadership and commitment to these methods are experiencing success, improving patient safety, and supporting their staff in a learning environment.

SIX SIGMA

In addition to the Model for Improvement and Lean Methodology, organizations may want to consider using Six Sigma to achieve improvement. This is a multifaceted performance improvement strategy that focuses on making every step in a process as reliable as it can be. The scope of this publication does not allow an in-depth discussion of Six Sigma; however a brief overview is included here for reference.[4]

Six Sigma was heavily inspired by six preceding decades of quality improvement methodologies, such as Quality Control, Total Quality Management, and Zero Defects. Like its predecessors, Six Sigma asserts the following:

- Continuous effort to reduce variation in process outputs is key to success.
- Processes can be measured, analyzed, improved, and controlled.
- Succeeding at achieving sustained quality improvement requires commitment from the entire organization, particularly from top-level management.

The core of the Six Sigma methodology is a data-driven, systematic approach to problem solving, with a focus on customer impact. Statistical tools and analysis are often useful in the process. However, an acceptable Six Sigma project can be started with only rudimentary statistical tools.

Six Sigma has two key methodologies[5] both inspired by W. Edwards Deming's Plan-Do-Check-Act Cycle. The first methodology, Define-Measure-Analyze-Improve-Control (DMAIC), is used to improve an existing process. The steps involved in DMAIC are as follows:

- *Define* the process improvement goals.
- *Measure* the current process and collect relevant data for future comparison.
- *Analyze* to verify relationship and causality of factors. Determine what the relationship is and attempt to ensure that all factors have been considered.
- *Improve* or optimize the process based upon the analysis.
- *Control* to ensure that any variances are corrected before they result in defects.

The second methodology, Define-Measure-Analyze-Design-Verify (DMADV), is used to create highly reliable designs for new processes. The steps involved in DMADV are as follows:

- *Define* the goals of the design activity.
- *Measure* and identify critical qualities, process capabilities, and risk assessments.
- *Analyze* to develop and design alternatives, create high-level design, and evaluate design capability to select the best design.
- *Design* details, optimize the design, and plan for design verification. This phase may require simulations.
- *Verify* the design, set up pilot runs, implement the process, and hand over to process owners.

Six Sigma identifies several key roles for its successful implementation, as follows[6,7]:

- *Executive Leadership* is responsible for setting up a vision for Six Sigma implementation. They also empower the other role holders with the freedom and resources to explore new ideas for breakthrough improvements.
- *Champions* are responsible for the Six Sigma implementation across the organization in an integrated manner.
- *Master Black Belts*, identified by champions, act as in-house expert coaches for the organization on Six Ssigma.
- *Black Belts* operate under Master Black Belts to apply Six Sigma methodology to specific projects.
- *Green Belts* are the employees who take up Six Sigma implementation along with their other job responsibilities. They operate under the guidance of Black Belts and support them in achieving the overall results.
- *Yellow Belts* are employees who have been trained in Six Sigma techniques as part of a corporatewide initiative, but have not completed a Six Sigma project and are not expected to actively engage in quality improvement activities.

TOOLS FOR USE IN PERFORMANCE IMPROVEMENT

Key components to all the previously discussed improvement approaches are studying the process you want to improve, identifying areas of risk and waste, and determining opportunities for improvement. Two tools that can help with this effort are discussed below.

Failure Mode and Effects Analysis

Failure mode and effects analysis[4] (FMEA) is a team-based, systematic, *proactive* technique used to prevent problems before they occur. It analyzes potential failures of systems, components, or functions and their effects. Each component is considered in turn with its possible modes of failure defined and the potential defects delineated.[8] It provides a look not only at what problems could occur but also at how severe the effects of the problems could be. FMEA assumes that no matter how knowledgeable or careful people are, failures will occur in some situations and may even be likely to occur. The focus is on *what* could allow the failure to occur, rather than *whom*. The FMEA technique is based on studied engineering principles and approaches to designing systems and processes. It has been successfully used in a number of industries, including the airline, automotive, and aerospace industries. Varying by the source consulted, FMEA can involve from as few as 4 to as many as 10 different steps. The approach described below has 8 key steps, as follows[4]:

1. Select a high-risk process and assemble a team.
2. Describe the process.
3. Brainstorm potential failure modes and determine their effects.
4. Prioritize failure modes.
5. Identify root causes of failure modes.
6. Redesign the process.
7. Analyze and test the new process.
8. Implement and monitor the redesigned process.

When conducting an FMEA, teams should answer some questions, including the following:

• What are the steps in the process? If it is an existing process, how does it currently occur and how should it occur? If it is a new process, how should it occur?

• How are the steps interrelated? (For example, are they sequential or do they occur simultaneously?)

• How is the process related to other health care processes?

• What tools should be used to diagram the process?

• What is the manner in which this process could fail? (When answering this question, team members should consider how people, materials, equipment, other processes and procedures, and the environment affect the process.)

• What are the potential effects of the identified failures? Effects of failures might be direct or indirect; long- or short-term; or likely or unlikely to occur. The severity of effects can vary considerably, from a minor annoyance to death or permanent loss of function. In this part of the process, team members should think through all the possible effects of a failure and list them for reference.

• What are the root causes of prioritized failure modes? What would have to go wrong for a failure like this to happen? What underlying weaknesses in the system might allow this to happen? What safeguards (for example, double checks) are present in the process? Are there any missing? If the process already contains safeguards, why might they not work to prevent the failure every time? If this failure occurred, why would the problem not be identified before it affected a patient?

Root Cause Analysis

Another tool that can be helpful when further identifying and defining a problem or process to study is root cause analysis.[9] Root cause analysis (RCA) is a process for identifying the basic or causal factors that underlie variations in performance. Variations in performance can (and often do) produce unexpected and undesired adverse outcomes, including the occurrence or risk of a sentinel event.[4]

Like FMEA, an RCA focuses primarily on systems and processes, not on the performance of a particular person. Through RCA, a team works to understand a process or processes, the causes or potential causes of variation, and process changes that make variation less likely to occur in the future. Root cause analysis is most commonly used *reactively* to probe the reason for a bad outcome or for failures that have already occurred. It can also be used to probe a near miss event or as part of the FMEA process.

A thorough and credible root cause analysis has several steps. Many of the steps involved in RCA are similar to FMEA, and are as follows[4]:

1. Organize a team.
2. Define the problem.
3. Study the problem.
4. Determine what happened.
5. Identify the contributing factors.
6. Collect and assess data on proximate and underlying causes.
7. Design and implement interim changes.
8. Determine the root causes.
9. Explore and identify risk reduction strategies.
10. Evaluate proposed actions.
11. Design, test, and implement improvements.
12. Evaluate and communicate the results of improvements.

By using root cause analysis to dig deep and discover the primary system issues causing error(s), organizations can target improvement efforts to reach the areas that will have the greatest impact on safety.

REFERENCES

1. Institute for Healthcare Improvement: *How to Improve.* http://www.ihi.org/IHI/Topics/Improvement/ImprovementMethods/HowToImprove (accessed Jul. 1, 2008).

2. Rogers E.: *Diffusion of Innovations,* 4th ed. New York: The Free Press, 1995.

3. Liker J.: *The Toyota Way.* New York: McGraw-Hill, 2003.

4. Joint Commission Resources: *Managing Performance Measurement Data in Health Care,* 2nd ed. Oakbrook Terrace, IL: The Joint Commission, 2008.

5. De Feo J., Barnard W.: *JURAN Institute's Six Sigma Breakthrough and Beyond—Quality Performance Breakthrough Methods. Mumbai:* Tata McGraw-Hill Publishing Company Limited, 2005.

6. Harry M., Schroeder R: *Six Sigma.* New York: Random House, 2000.

7. Motorola University. *Six Sigma Dictionary.* http://www.motorola.com/content.jsp?globalObjectId=3074-5804 (accessed Jul. 10, 2008).

8. Vincent C.: Human error assessment and reduction technique, HEART Patient Safety. Edinburgh: Elsevier, 2006.

9. National Center for Patient Safety: *Root Cause Analysis (RCA).* http://www.va.gov/NCPS/rca.html (accessed Oct. 30, 2008).

Chapter Thirteen

PRACTICAL ASPECTS OF IMPLEMENTATION

Michael Leonard, Allan Frankel, Michael Fox, Terri Simmonds, **and** *Carol Haraden*

Safety and reliability in health care are both possible and necessary. Throughout this book, we have discussed that the journey toward safety and reliability requires unrelenting and committed leadership, transparency about error, and consistent, effective teamwork and communication. While the previous chapters have introduced concepts that are necessary to achieve a safe and reliable system for health care, this chapter focuses on taking these concepts and applying them within your organization. The first part of the chapter introduces a recommended sequence for action, and the second part focuses on implementing recommendations for specific areas of health care.

SEQUENCING FOR ACTION

Understanding the concepts behind safety culture, accountability, high reliability, teamwork and communication, disclosure, patient involvement, and process improvement are important, but when you finish reading this book, how are you going to take all this information and start? Do you know where to begin? The following sequence is recommended based on the collective opinions, research, and tested theories of the contributors to this book. By following this sequence you can create a clear path toward high reliability, enhanced safety, improved quality of care, and exceptional performance. (Table 13-1 on pages 114–115 provides a time line that organizations can also follow to help with implementation.)

Step 1: Engage leaders, both senior and physician, around transparency and continuous learning. This will involve creating an accountability system and a systematic flow of information. Senior and clinical leaders must commit resources to safety culture assessment, teamwork training, direct observation, and establishing a steering com-

mittee to drive the work. They must be crystal clear on an organizationwide commitment to safety, accept no exceptions, and deal consistently with providers who "don't want to play".

Step 2: Systematically survey the culture and identify areas of risk. Look at the results of safety culture surveys and connect these results to inherently high-risk clinical areas—obstetrics (OB), surgery, emergency medicine, medical/surgical units with high rates of patients requiring acute intervention—and your own clinical events, both near misses and sentinel events. Also use a cyclic flow of information from Executive WalkRounds™, spontaneous reporting, and glitch books to inform where the greatest opportunities for improvement are, both with regard to culture and processes of care.

Step 3: Provide targeted team training that combines specific tools and behaviors, which are embedded within clinical domain-specific processes of care. Engage leadership support, have a steering group of champions to support and drive the work, and have specific measures that offer feedback and demonstrate improvement. Realize that cultural change is behavior over time, and by far the most effective results come from organizations that invest in multidisciplinary team training—physicians, nurses, tech- nicians, and other personnel in the room together learning, practicing teamwork and tools, and building social agreement as to how they will work together.

Step 4: Reliably design processes. Reach agreement on clinical measures that are important and relevant to the clinical area. Have the teams define the system issues that get in the way of optimal care. A useful way to have this conversation is to have the team define optimal care, and then discuss the things that get in the way of that goal. Now the group

Table 13-1. Time Line for Implementation

Stage 1: Team Training
Stage 2: Spread Across Organization

Month	Name	Description–Heart Institute
0	Phone Conference Calls	*Telephone Conference Calls.* Discuss with senior leadership the resources needed for cultural assessment, the leadership engagement required, and the use of the data to direct improvement activity.
1–3	Cultural Assessment Using Safety Attitudes Questionnaire (SAQ)	Perform Cultural Assessment using Safety Attitudes Questionnaire for entire unit or department.
3	Phone Conference Call	Analyze SAQ results with senior leadership. Identify areas for further analysis (to be performed on site through focused interviews) and, based on SAQ results, improvement work to be performed.
3	Phone Conference Call	Conference call with Clinical Leaders.
4	Site Visit (4 days)	**Day 1: Focused Interviews:** Focused interviews based on SAQ findings (to further enhance cultural assessment and focus training for next three days) **Day 2 and 3: Foundations:** Improvement and Teamwork. Each department participating in these two days chooses a team of 3 to 6 individuals. Team members should represent the disciplines in the unit, include physicians and nurses, have one senior or departmental leader, and be chosen for interest and willingness to test changes and improve. There can be up to 200 people in total. Prework for two days is to identify areas for improvement in their units. Ideally, if some problems are at department interfaces, teams across the interface would be paired and be jointly responsible for both teams' improvement efforts. On day 2, teams would learn improvement methods and then apply them to their specific issues. On day 3 teams would learn teamwork components and begin to consider application of some teamwork components appropriate for their units. The latter part of day 3 would be linking teamwork and improvement concepts into a cohesive plan for each departmental team. **Day 4: Concurrent Sessions** 1. Foundations—Focused team training overview (concurrent sessions)–Two departments (to be chosen); introduce teamwork and improvement concepts in two 4-hour sessions for 2 units including entire staff of units. During these sessions, clinical activity would need to stop or be significantly curtailed. 2. Observation Training (concurrent sessions)—Small cohort of clinicians would be trained specifically in observation in interventional areas (ideally, same units involved in **Focused team training**).
5–15	1 Hour/Month Conference Calls	Conference call with departmental teams to discuss projects—successes and hurdles.
6	1 Hour Conference Call	Spread plans. Discuss how to take learning from units participating in team training and spread to other areas of organization.

(continued on page 115)

Table 13-1. Time Line for Implementation (continued)

Month	Name	Description–Heart Institute
8–12 (Date to be chosen based on how fast teams get up to speed with their work. If struggling, plan for Month 7; if doing well, plan for Month 10.)	Site Visit 4 Days	**Day 1: Observation training** for 2–4 new sites. Begin baseline observation in the 2–4 identified sites. Focused interviews. **Day 2: All Team Retreat**—Showcase projects and work performed. Revisit and expand on improvement skills. **Day 3: Champion Training**—Work with selected group to assist in training 2–4 new units in team training. **Day 4: Foundations**—Focused team training overview: Introduce teamwork and improvement concepts in two 4-hour sessions for 2–4 units including entire staff of units. During these sessions, clinical activity would need to stop or be significantly curtailed.
14–16		Repeat SAQ.
14	Conference Call	Discuss site visit plans and next steps. (that is, simulation training to support teamwork efforts)
18	Site Visit 2 days	Facilitate two-day collaborative meeting of safety champions from all departments. Review internal teamwork, clinical and interface successes and issues. Plan next steps.

This table shows a sample time line organizations can follow to help guide implementation efforts.

Source: Allan Frankel. Used with permission.

has defined their performance gap. Choose two or three areas to start working on. By clearly focusing on a few areas, measuring and improving, the teams will build a critical skill, namely the capacity to do process improvement well. This learning can be applied to future areas of improvement.

Step 5: Apply direct observation and feedback to observe teamwork behaviors and monitor the success of initiatives. To do this effectively, build the organizational capacity to do this well. Baseline observation combined with safety culture data is a very powerful way to engage a clinical area in the value of effective teamwork and clinical improvement. Measure postintervention and at ongoing intervals to sustain and track progress.

Step 6: Define, implement, monitor, and establish a feedback mechanism for process, outcome, and organizational measures to show success and drive improvement. Process measures show whether the processes of care were followed (patients received timely antibiotics before surgery 100% of the time); outcome measures look at clinical outcomes (how many patients had unplanned returns to the operating room after surgery); and organizational measures

reflect system issues (how often surgical cases were started on time). Effective feedback is timely, is related to clinical work frontline caregivers see as important, and reflects the improvement that teams have accomplished. Caregivers are both busy and dedicated; show them their work is making a difference in how patients are cared for.

Step 7: Use performance improvement strategies to structure continuous improvement. Teach tools and build capacity to do this work. It is essential that busy clinicians and leaders can see that the work being done creates value for patients, the organization, and the people doing the work. Having the ability to widely share information about improvement, and being able to spread it to other clinical areas, is essential.

While each step in the sequence is unique, you do not completely finish one step before starting another. In this case, each step builds upon the previous step, so by the end of the sequence you are continuously pursing all seven steps at the same time. Think of it like learning to walk. Although you first learn to balance, then to stand, and then to take a tentative step, you don't forget those initial skills but use them in an integrated process that helps move you forward. In the same vein, you don't engage leadership, assess teamwork, or define performance measures just once; you do them all simultaneously as you move toward safe and reliable care.

IMPLEMENTATION STRATEGIES FOR DIFFERENT SETTINGS

Although the need for safe care is apparent in all settings of health care, there are several areas that present higher risks for error and patient harm because of the nature of the care provided in these settings, the acuity of patient illness, the unpredictability of patient volume, the time frame necessary for adequate care, the players involved in the care, or the structure of the system that supports the care. This section takes a look at some of these areas and provides strategies for improving safety and reliability.

Operating Room (OR)

Successful communication in the OR is dependent upon team leadership setting the appropriate tone, using structured communication techniques, establishing and reinforcing red rules *see* page 118 in this chapter), and fostering an environment of learning and performance improvement.[1-6]

When beginning work in the OR, you must designate a clinical leadership group that will own and drive the work. Without such designated leadership keeping surgical improvement as a "front-burner" issue, providers will revert to previous thinking and the gains can become diffused. Such leaders must be committed to safety, able to drive cultural change, and willing to occasionally participate in some difficult conversations.

Assess the Culture of the OR

After leadership is engaged, they should review the cultural assessment information about the OR. As described in Chapter 2, cultural assessments are most valuable when done at the unit level, so your organization should have ready information about cultural attitudes in the OR by service line. In addition, leaders may want to conduct a quick mini–mental assessment of the culture. Such a mini-assessment—a "social apgar™" of sorts—can help verify safety culture of the unit and gauge the tone of the room, interaction between care providers, and the perspective of

patients. When conducting a social apgar consider the following three areas:

1. Safety culture—as a nurse or physician, what does it feel like to be in the room? Is there open communication, do providers feel comfortable speaking up; is there psychological safety; are problems worked through constructively?[7]

2. Patient satisfaction—what is the level of patient satisfaction with the care in the unit? Are patients pleased and do they believe that patient care teams communicate well? As discussed in Chapter 9, ineffective communication and poor teamwork are not lost on the patient. As they receive care, patients notice whether physicians and nurses interact effectively or work at odds with one another. They sense hostility, resentment, and confusion. Considering the patient perspective is critical. If patients are not happy with what they see, you are not going to be successful in a competitive market. By considering their perspective, you may identify problems you didn't even know you had.[8]

3. Nursing turnover—are nursing providers voting with their feet in this unit? Does this indicate a deeper issue? It is important to note that for organizations that have a high-performance culture based on teamwork and communication, such as the Dana-Farber Cancer Institute, there is very little nursing turnover.[9] However, other organizations can turn over up to 25% of their nurses per year. What does this say about the culture of these organizations? Replacing nurses is expensive and wasteful. It is very hard to achieve consistent, high-level team performance and deliver safe care without workforce stability.

A social apgar can be done in places other than just the OR and can help leaders take the pulse and temperature of the organization and identify areas where teamwork and communication need to improve. Performing a social apgar on each unit can also help identify potential risk. Consider units that are inherently high risk because of the types of procedures, patients, and interventions performed, such as the intensive care unit (ICU), emergency department, operating room, and labor and delivery unit. Consider both the near misses and sentinel events in these areas as well as the social apgar on these units. If a unit has high risk for error and a low social apgar, this can reveal an area of high risk, and the unit should go to the top of the list for areas that need improvement.

Provide Teamwork Training

Nowhere is teamwork training more critical and more necessary than the OR. Surgeons are trained to be individual experts, relying on themselves to deliver high-quality care.[10] It is essential, in fact imperative, to regularly have multidisciplinary teamwork training sessions for this area, which involve nurses, surgeons, anesthesiologists, technicians, and other members of the care team. As previously discussed, such training should involve storytelling—related to real clinical events—to reemphasize critical messages and scenarios, which allow teams to practice working together.

Team training should include drills in which team members practice for emergency scenarios to ensure that teamwork behaviors and communication strategies continue during high-stress, emergency situations. There is great value in simulation, both high- and low-tech approaches.

Use Structured Communication Techniques

While many structured communication tools are critical to enhancing safety in the OR—active callouts, Situation, Background, Assessment, Recommendation (SBAR), effective assertion/critical language, and so forth—one of the most important tools is the briefing.[11] With a preprocedure briefing the surgeon sets the tone for the procedure in the first moments of the team coming together, shares the plan, and continuously invites the other team members into the conversation both for their expertise and concerns. While clearly in charge, surgeons must be approachable, encourage feedback, respond respectfully to questions and concerns, and promote an atmosphere of collaboration and problem solving.[12] This briefing can be as short as 45 seconds and still establish an environment of collaboration and teamwork if the surgeon shares the plan, possible contingencies, and possible risk points. The surgeon should use people's first names and invite them specifically to provide feedback. It's important when sharing the plan that the conversation is not unidirectional. Saying, "Let me tell you how this is going to work" will not establish the right tone. Instead, "Here's what we're doing today and here's what I'm thinking about the process. Do we have the right tools? Information? What are the potential problems? Does anyone have any thoughts, questions, or concerns?"

In addition, briefings in the OR should occur on the spot, as conditions change, and during patient handoffs. Team leaders need to quickly brief new team members as people take breaks or change shifts. Ideally, a briefing should also take place when a patient is scheduled for surgery to anticipate equipment and supply needs.

As mentioned in Chapter 6 on page 53, The Joint Commission requires organizations to conduct preprocedure briefings as part of its Universal Protocol for Preventing Wrong Site, Wrong Procedure, Wrong Person Surgery™. Along the same lines, the World Health Organization recently rolled out a surgical safety checklist that can be helpful in OR briefings. (*See* Figure 13-1 on page 118.) This checklist stages the briefing process and encourages effective communication and team behaviors throughout surgery.

Critical language is essential in a high-risk environment like the OR. The ability to say "I need a little clarity" and have the team stop and ensure that they are going the right direction is very important. Knowing the plan makes it much easier to ask for clarity. Active callouts where the team thinks out loud—"we're closing"—and thinks ahead—"we'll need radiology in about 30 minutes"—are very valuable. Teams that think out loud and anticipate contingencies maintain situational awareness and are able to mentally rehearse clinical challenges. In de Leval's cardiac surgery work, the teams exhibiting these behaviors had better clinical outcomes.[13]

Debriefing is also a very valuable activity.[4] Take one to two minutes at the end of the case—while waking the patient up or putting the dressing on—and capture information while it is fresh in everyone's minds. The basic aspect of debriefing is that everyone contributes, beginning with the most junior team members, so they won't be overly influenced by the senior team members. The debriefing is always framed to the positive—"what did we learn, what did we do well, what will we do differently the next time, etc.?" Coupling the debriefing with a glitch book to collect, track and feed back the improvement ideas is essential (*see* below).

Some other effective communication tools to use in the OR include the following:

• The Glitch Book. As discussed in Chapter 5, this tool helps communicate issues discovered at the unit level up to leadership. Such a tool can be helpful in ensuring that issues that come up in surgery—faulty equipment, supply shortages, concerns about staffing—are addressed in a timely manner. It is essential that members of the OR team believe that if they point out a flaw in the process of care, that someone listens every time and fixes the problem if possible.

Figure 13-1. Surgical Safety Checklist

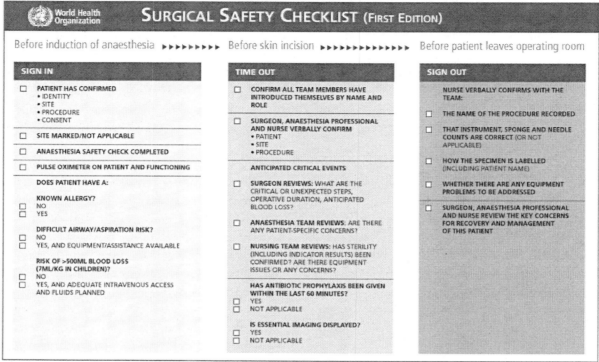

This checklist was recently developed by the World Health Organization to help structure communication in the operating room.

Source: World Health Organization. Used with permission.

Without a systematic feedback and improvement loop, providers stop speaking up.

• **Whiteboards.** Whiteboards are an effective tool to help with situational awareness. Information included on the whiteboard should include the names of all surgical team members, a description of the process, the name of the patient, and special equipment or tests.

• **Red Rules.** As discussed in Chapter 6, these are mandatory rules that everyone agrees must be followed every time. Surgery has two critical red rules:

1. Always verify the correct site, procedure, and patient before incision—every time.

2. If there is a count discrepancy with regard to sponges or instruments, you never leave the OR without an x-ray.

Performance Measure for the OR

There are several critical measures that help ensure performance in the OR, including but not limited to, the following:

• Surgical Care Improvement Project (SCIP) measures required by the Centers for Medicare & Medicaid. These include measures about glucose levels, prophylactic antibiotics, appropriate beta blockers, deep venous thrombosis prophylaxis, discontinuing antibiotics after 24 hours, and so forth.

• Triggers that indicate a potential adverse event. As described in Chapter 5, these can include an unplanned return to surgery, reintubation, and transfusion.

• Operational measures, such as percentage of on-time starts, cancellations, delays, intraoperative delays (rarely captured, but very common), OR turnover, and equipment glitches.

Obstetrics and Gynecology

The obstetrics department of a hospital is truly a complex system, and all the risks associated with such a system can be present on any given day. Safety in obstetrics (OB) requires the following:

- Strong and engaged team leadership
- Regular safety culture assessment and feedback
- Effective communication and teamwork training (Do this in multidisciplinary groups.)
- Common language to describe fetal heart tracings. The National Institute of Child Health and Human Development (NICHD) has developed standardized and unambiguous definitions for fetal heart rate (FHR) tracings that are to be used in all professional and written communications in the obstetric setting. By systematically using NICHD terminology, you improve the likelihood that both the deliverer and recipient of information about a FHR tracing will base their interventions on an accurate and shared understanding of the state of the FHR tracing at any given moment.
- Use a common interpretive construct to evaluate fetal heart tracings. Michael Fox and colleagues from the University of California, San Francisco, created a systemized approach to monitoring and interpreting fetal heart tracings. This system provides a good example of how a simple, shared, and systematic approach to FHR tracing interpretation and management can help providers predetermine relative priorities, and effectively focus a team's attention to high-priority observations and interventions.[14] (*See* Appendix beginning on page 127 for more information on Fox's work.)
- Use multidisciplinary rounds, which include obstetricians, midwives, nurses, technicians, and other personnel. A representative from anesthesia and the neonatal intensive care unit (NICU) is highly desirable. Such rounds should occur at the beginning of the shift, with brief, rapid updates periodically throughout the shift to highlight risky patients, assess workflow, and reconfirm patient care plans. While low-risk patients may be discussed only briefly, it is important to talk about the care of each patient as two thirds of obstetrical disasters happen in low-risk patients because everyone assumes the patient will be fine, and staff members are often hesitant to bring up problems when they surface. Within these multidisciplinary rounds, all participants must feel comfortable speaking up and be specifically invited to do so. Because an OB provider's workload is unpredictable at times, it is also important that when someone believes they are getting behind or overwhelmed, that he or she is empowered and in fact required to quickly get the team back together and reassess the workload.

- Create a red rule for physician response. As previously mentioned, an important red rule for obstetrics is when someone is concerned at the bedside and asks a clinician to come to the bedside, he or she should come 100% of the time. It is essential that the physician respond in a timely and respectful fashion. If not, the provider making the request, who is clearly interested in doing what is best for the patient, may be more hesitant in the future to seek help.
- Create a red rule for social inductions. When a baby is induced prior to 39 weeks for social reasons, there is increased risk to the health of the baby and the mother. By creating a red rule, organizations underscore the importance of not inducing electively prior to 39 weeks for nonmedical reasons. Many leading hospital systems have eliminated social inductions prior to 39 weeks.
- Ensure consistency regarding Pitocin administration. Do you have one or two Pitocin protocols (low-dose and high-dose, for example) that clearly state the dose and timing of when to increase or decrease the Pitocin, by how much, and at what intervals? In most hospitals, this is not the case, and the dose and time frames for increasing Pitocin differ significantly from physician to physician. This requires nurses within these organizations to be familiar with multiple protocols for administering Pitocin. This sets up a situation ripe for error and harm and sends the message that the personality of the providers and their personal experience, not collectively determined guidelines, determines how and in what way Pitocin will be administered. Organizations should design a protocol for Pitocin administration that standardizes the process and ensures reliability.
- Have standardized approaches to shoulder dystocias, practice them, and debrief.
- Develop a standardized approach to vacuum extractions—answering the question how many times can you "pop-off" and how long can you persist before everyone knows you move to Plan B? This is really important, as practitioners can get task fixated in stressful situations and persist far longer than is in anyone's interest. It's much easier for the nurse or someone else in the room to say "we have exceeded our agreed limit, we need to go down the hall now" than to try to determine the appropriate approach on the fly.
- Practice for emergencies. Effective communication and teamwork in stressful situations will not reliably occur unless it is practiced. To do this in OB, teams should engage in drills or videotaped simulations with feedback. These sim-

ulations allow members of the OB team to assess whether their communication is effective. The simulations also help team members identify important logistical, environmental, and resource issues. These scenario drills should focus on situations commonly associated with emergent delivery and maternal care—such as shoulder dsytocias and vacuum extractions—but can also address low occurrence catastrophes such as a cardiac arrest in the bed, umbilical cord prolapsed, or amniotic fluid embolism, which require emergently moving to the OR.

• Use clinical metrics, process redesign, and feedback to drive improvement.

Measures for OB

A key measure for OB is the adverse perinatal outcomes index or the Institute for Healthcare Improvement (IHI) Perinatal Trigger Tool. This helps determine how often things go awry in the department and areas of teamwork, communication, and reliability system development that need improvement. Another effective measure is event to delivery time. This looks at the time frame between an emergency, such as an acute drop in blood pressure, and the time the baby is delivered. By monitoring this measure you can see if initiatives to promote effective communication during an emergency, team training, and emergency drills are effective.

Emergency Department (ED)

As with the OB department, ED staff cannot control how many patients enter the ED at any given time. For that reason alone, structured communication techniques, multi-disciplinary rounds, briefings, and red rules are important, not to mention because of the complex procedures that occur in the ED and the critical nature of the patients treated there. In addition, reliability is often weak in the ED as providers don't consistently "do the basics" in responding to high-risk diagnoses, and sometimes unstable patients can be sent home only to collapse in the parking lot. In addition, long wait times can cause people to leave without being seen, and patients can decompensate while waiting for an inpatient bed.

To help ensure reliability and safety in the ED, consider the following interventions:

• Identify a discrete list of high-risk diagnoses and standardize the care associated with those processes to ensure that the basics of care are provided every time. Such stan-

dardization could involve a checklist and a protocol that empowers anyone to "stop the line" if items on the checklist are skipped.

• Assign the most expert person to do triage. Often triage is delegated down to the least experienced person because it is the least desirable job. However, from a patient safety perspective, your organization should have someone who has experience in providing patient care to do triage as he or she can better differentiate the seriousness of problems and steer the patient toward the appropriate care. This not only helps ensure that the right care is given, but it also helps flow through the ED. By efficiently and effectively getting patients the care they need, it can prevent unnecessary delays and rework.

• Establish a fast track or urgent care unit. This helps separate urgent fixable problems from emergent ones that require intense resources, such as provider time and equipment, that will most probably lead to inpatient admission. Such units can help reduce patient wait times, ensure reliability of care, and improve resource utilization. Ideally, fast track units should be physically separated from the regular ED to help with patient flow and infection control issues.

• Fast-track lab, radiology, pharmacy results, and prescriptions. In the ED, a quick turnaround on laboratory reports, X-rays, and medications is essential for safe care and patient satisfaction. It doesn't do any good to get a patient in a room quickly if you don't have medications or test results to assess. Likewise, patient satisfaction will be affected if the patient is waiting 40 minutes for a prescription just so he or she can go home. The ED should work with the laboratory, radiology, and pharmacy departments to fast-track results and prescriptions to ensure prompt, reliable care.

• Create a protocol whereby patients who have been admitted to the hospital but who remain in the ED waiting for an inpatient bed are reexamined by an ED physician every two hours. In some facilities, 30% of people who are admitted to the hospital remain in the ED for a long period of time. Because the patient could start to decline, someone should reevaluate them periodically.

Some areas to measure that show performance in the ED include compliance with checklists for high-risk diagnoses, ED throughput, and abandonment.

Intensive Care Unit (ICU)

As with other settings, strong clinical leadership, teamwork behaviors and communication techniques, such as SBAR, briefings, and multidisciplinary rounds, are critical in this environment. Because of the intense nature of the care delivered and the potential hierarchies that exist in this setting, it is also critical to continuously reassess the safety culture of the ICU. As with the OR, using a "social apgar" can help determine issues that need to be addressed.

In addition to instilling, training, and reinforcing teamwork behaviors, other process interventions to pursue in the ICU include the following:

• Implement a process for creating and rounding on daily goals. Organizations may want to create a daily goals form, which lists the tasks to be completed, the care plan, and the communication plan for discussions with the patient, and his or her family, for a particular day.[15] A variety of questions should be addressed on this form, including, "What needs to be done for the patient to be discharged from the ICU?" and "What is the patient's greatest safety risk, and how can we decrease risk?"[16]

• Develop systematic and standardized processes to consistently address critical issues, such as ventilator-associated pneumonia (VAP) and central line infections (CLI). Organizations should measure compliance with the processes to ensure consistent and appropriate care. The IHI recommends several standardized interventions to address VAP[17], including the following:

—Ventilator-associated pneumonia

 ○ Elevate the head of the bed.

 ○ Perform daily "sedation vacations" and assessment of readiness to extubate.

 ○ Implement peptic ulcer disease prophylaxis.

 ○ Implement deep venous thrombosis prophylaxis.

More information about the VAP bundle can be found at http://www.ihi.org.

When considering how to achieve safe and reliable care with regard to central line infections, look at the state of Michigan's Keystone ICU project in reducing catheter-related bloodstream infections. Because of the health care system in the state of Michigan, 103 ICUs participated in the project.

To reduce infections, the ICUs implemented the following five evidence-based procedures that are recommended by the Centers for Disease Control and Prevention and identified as having the greatest effect on the rate of catheter-related bloodstream infection and the lowest barri-

ers to implementation.

• Hand washing

• Using full-barrier precautions during the insertion of central venous catheters

• Cleaning the skin with chlorhexidine

• Avoiding the femoral site

• Removing unnecessary catheters as soon as feasible

The key element in the project, however, was not the procedures but the teamwork piece. Each ICU designated at least one physician and one nurse to be team leaders for the project. These individuals were instructed in the science of safety and trained via weekly conference calls, research staff coaching, and statewide meetings twice a year. The teams received supporting information on the efficacy of each component of the intervention, suggestions for implementing each component, and instruction in methods of data collection. Team leaders partnered with their local hospital-based infection control practitioners to assist in the implementation of the intervention and to obtain data on catheter-related bloodstream infections at the hospital. Team leaders educated clinicians about practices to control infection and harm resulting from catheter-related bloodstream infections.

In addition to the focus on teamwork, the ICUs engaged in the following actions:

• Created a central line cart with necessary supplies

• Used a checklist to ensure adherence to infection control practices

• Consistently stopped providers (in nonemergency situations) if these practices were not being followed

• Discussed the removal of catheters during daily rounds

One interesting aspect of the project involved the use of chlorhexidine. In April 2004 a letter and a baseline survey were sent to the CEOs of the participating hospitals. The letter outlined the evidence supporting the use of chlorhexidine and asked the CEOs to stock chlorhexidine in their hospitals before implementing the study intervention. Across the board, senior leaders made the decision to stock chlorhexidine.

Teams received feedback regarding the number and rates of catheter-related bloodstream infection at monthly and quarterly meetings, respectively. Before the project began, ICUs in the state of Michigan experienced 2.7 infections per 1,000 catheter-days. Three months after implementation the central line infection rate across the entire state decreased 70%, which translated to more than a thousand saved lives and a couple of hundred million dollars of avoided cost. The benefit was maintained at that level even 16–18 months after implementation. This example shows that with strong commitment, effective teamwork, reliable processes, and regular communication, organizations can achieve great things.[18]

Medical/Surgical Units (Med/Surg)

As with all the previously discussed settings, safe care in the med/surg area involves strong leadership, effective teamwork, and reliable processes. Specific interventions that are critical to this area include the following:

• Designate a physician to "own" the patient. Within the medical/surgical environment, patients have many different clinicians, specialists, technologists, and so forth that handle their care. When there is a question about a patient, often the nurse does not know who to call and may waste precious time hunting down a physician. This is not only a waste of time but presents a patient safety issue as it may take several minutes to hours to identify the correct provider. To address this, organizations must have a process in which a specific physician serves as the primary point of contact for each patient. In many cases this is a hospitalist; however, within organizations without hospitalists, another option is necessary. (*See* Sidebar 13-1, right.)

• Nurses and physicians need to round together. This ensures that everyone is on the same page about the patient's care. Information to cover within the rounding process includes the following:

—What's the overall plan of care? What is the specific plan for today?

—What issues should the nurse watch out for? What are the triggers to call and ask for help?

—Who should the nurse call for help?

—Who is the designated physician that "owns" the patient?

—When do we need to increase the intensity of care and recruit help?

• Create a rapid response team (RRT). This is a team of clinicians who bring critical-care expertise to the patient bedside quickly and willingly to assess the patient and then recommend or undertake interventions. This group can respond when other hospital caregivers believe a patient is

---

Sidebar 13-1. Solving the Geography Problem

A hospitalist is a designated physician who works full-time in the hospital. Because they are always on site, they are a logical solution to the medical/surgical problem of "who owns the patient." However, even with the use of hospitalists, organizations need to solve the "geography problem." In many organizations a hospitalist is responsible for patients across many different floors. He or she spends valuable time running between units and does not develop productive relationships with the nursing staff. Some organizations are addressing this issue by committing to having 90% of a hospitalist's patients located on the same floor. This allows him or her to build better relationships with nurses and improve team performance.

---

showing signs of clinical deterioration. The goal of an RRT is not to take away a physician's or nurse's patient management responsibilities; rather, the focus is to quickly do what is required to prevent further worsening of the patient's condition and to avoid an arrest. In an Australian hospital where the RRT concept was first introduced, the hospital saw a 65% reduction in hospital cardiac arrest and a 24% reduction in overall hospital mortality.[19] Through the National Patient Safety Goals, The Joint Commission requires hospitals and critical access hospitals to improve recognition and response to changes in a patient's condition. One way to comply with this goal is to implement an RRT. (*See* Sidebar 13-2 on page 124 for more information about RRTs.)

• Create an early warning scoring system (EWSS). This is a way of documenting patient vital signs so that abnormal vital signs trigger a call to the RRT. Some organizations use a form as their EWSS. This form highlights problematic vital signs in red. If the individual taking the vital signs—often a nursing assistant—notes that a vital sign is in the red area, he or she knows to immediately call the nurse and/or the rapid response team. (*See* Figure 13-2 on page 123 for an example of such a form.) OSF Healthcare has automated its EWSS, so that when problematic vital signs are entered into the organization's computerized medical record, a warning flashes, prompting the nurse to call the RRT.[20]

Measuring Performance in Med/Surg

There are several measures that can help show perfor-

Figure 13-2. Vital Sign Documentation Tool

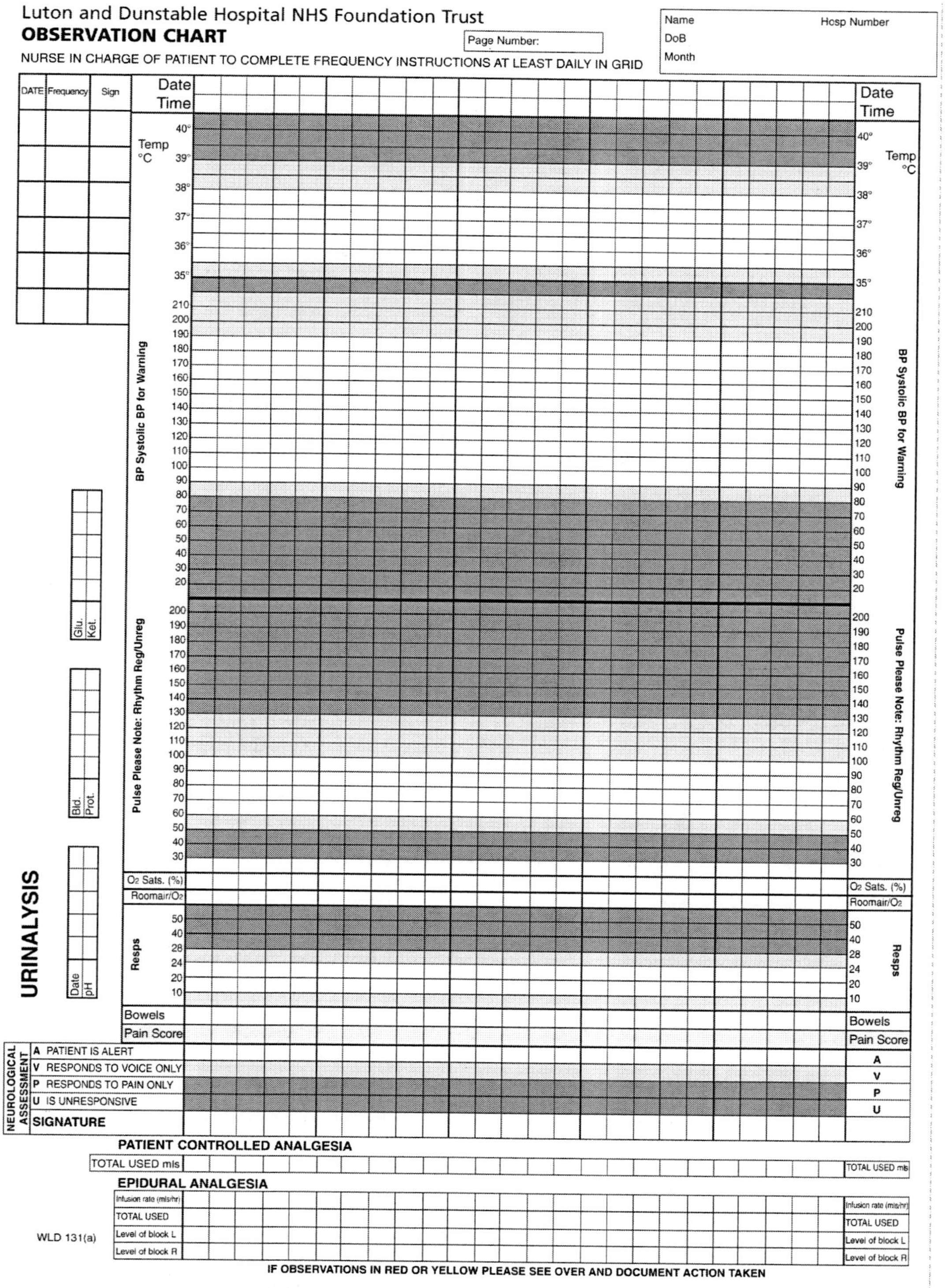
Luton and Dunstable Hospital NHS Foundation Trust
OBSERVATION CHART
Page Number:
NURSE IN CHARGE OF PATIENT TO COMPLETE FREQUENCY INSTRUCTIONS AT LEAST DAILY IN GRID
Name
Hosp Number
DoB
Month
DATE | Frequency | Sign
Date
Time
Temp °C 40° 39° 38° 37° 36° 35°
BP Systolic BP for Warning 210 200 190 180 170 160 150 140 130 120 110 100 90 80 70 60 50 40 30 20
Pulse Please Note: Rhythm Reg/Unreg 200 190 180 170 160 150 140 130 120 110 100 90 80 70 60 50 40 30
O2 Sats. (%)
Roomair/O2
Resps 50 40 28 24 20 10
Bowels
Pain Score
URINALYSIS
Glu.
Ket.
Bld.
Prot.
Date
pH
NEUROLOGICAL ASSESSMENT
A PATIENT IS ALERT
V RESPONDS TO VOICE ONLY
P RESPONDS TO PAIN ONLY
U IS UNRESPONSIVE
SIGNATURE
A
V
P
U
PATIENT CONTROLLED ANALGESIA
TOTAL USED mls
EPIDURAL ANALGESIA
Infusion rate (mls/hr)
TOTAL USED
Level of block L
Level of block R
WLD 131(a)
IF OBSERVATIONS IN RED OR YELLOW PLEASE SEE OVER AND DOCUMENT ACTION TAKEN

This paper-based tool can help clearly indicate when vital signs warrant a call to the rapid response team.

Source: Luton and Dunstable Hospital. Used with permission.

Sidebar 13-2. Rapid Response Teams

A rapid response team (RRT) is typically made up of a hospitalist or intensivist, intensive care unit (ICU) nurses, and a respiratory therapist. The purpose of the team is to get expertise to the bedside within 3–4 minutes every time there is a concern. Although criteria vary slightly from hospital to hospital, the following represent a common set of criteria that prompt a call to the RRT:

- Staff member is worried about the patient.
- Acute change in heart rate to < 40 or > 130 beats/minute
- Acute change in systolic blood pressure to < 90 mmHG
- Acute change in respiratory rate to < 8 or > 30 breaths/minute
- Acute change in pulse oximetry saturation to < 90% despite oxygen administration
- Acute change in conscious state
- Acute change in urine output to < 50 mL in four hours

Organizations that have an RRT encourage anyone—clinicians, patients, families, and so forth—to call upon the team whenever the patient meets certain criteria. These criteria are posted throughout the hospital, on medical/surgical units, in staff break rooms, and so forth.

Upon arriving at a patient's bedside, the role of the RRT is to do the following:

- Assess the patient. The RRT works to identify the problem by discussing the patient's condition with the staff member who called the team, evaluating the symptom(s) that prompted the call, examining and questioning the patient to learn more about the symptom(s), and reviewing the patient's chart for any other potential causes of the problem.
- Stabilize the patient. After the patient's problem has been identified, the RRT may follow preestablished clinical protocols that allow team members to quickly treat and/or stabilize the patient.
- Assist with communication among different care providers. RRT members will work with nursing staff and others to prepare the necessary communication to inform the attending physician, hospitalist, and/or primary care physician about the event.
- Educate and support the staff caring for the patient. By going over the call with the nurse (or other staff member providing care), the RRT members can educate the nurse about critical-care issues and provide vital information that will aid in future care decisions about that patient.
- Assist with transferring the patient to a higher level of care, such as the ICU, when necessary. If the patient's condition requires greater care, RRT members will assist the staff in the appropriate procedures for having that patient transferred to a monitored bed or the ICU.

Ideally, organizations build time for their RRTs to round on patient floors before they are called for an emergency. This allows them to get to know the nurses on the floor, proactively discuss any patients the nurses are concerned about, and lower the threshold for nurses to call them in the event of a concern. If not implemented with an emphasis on teamwork, frontline staff may be hesitant to call the RRT for fear of looking stupid. By rounding ahead of time, the team can reinforce the importance of calling them whenever there is a concern. Basically, the message should be, there is no bad time to call. If you are concerned, just call. To further reinforce this message, RRT members must always show up to a call with a smile on their face and a willingness to help the patient and provider. If the provider calls the RRT, and they express irritation for being called, or make the provider feel inadequate, that will quickly squelch the likelihood that the provider will call again.

By creating a specific team to respond to these issues, organizations can help get patients the care they need when they need it.[21] Because of the nursing shortage, more and more hospitals are hiring inexperienced nurses to work in more critical areas. The RRT brings an experienced nurse to the bedside in times of need and also helps further educate the unit nurse.

---

mance in medical/surgical units. For example, looking at clusters of rapid response calls, nursing turnover, patient satisfaction, the percentage of patients discharged by 11 A.M., and the consistency of discharge planning and education can identify areas of improvement. Within most health care organizations, there may be certain units that are at higher risk for adverse events. These units may have poor teamwork, lack of psychological safety, or other issues that need addressing. You should look at internal data to see if there are "high risk" spots in particular units. For example, if there are clusters of patients deteriorating unexpectedly on certain units that signals a problem. If there are a greater number of unanticipated adverse events on certain units, that signals a problem. Leaders may want to conduct a social apgar on those units. As previously mentioned, areas with high rates of adverse events and low social apgar could represent good locations to target improvement work.

Ambulatory Care

There are some unique challenges to the outpatient setting. Patients are in and out of facilities, and care is difficult to coordinate across providers. For this reason, strong teamwork and communication skills and reliable processes are critical for this setting. Following is a brief discussion of some of the initiatives that can improve safety in this area:

• Conduct regular briefings and debriefings. As discussed in Chapter 6, conducting regular briefings is critical in ambulatory care. Having one briefing in the morning to look ahead at the schedule and plan for patient care can identify information needs, ensure that everyone is on the same page, and give a sense of how the day will unfold. Team members can see the patients who will require more time, lab tests, and other interventions so they can plan ahead. In addition, touching base throughout the day can help reassess priorities, communicate new developments, and anticipate concerns. At the end of the day, team members should reconvene for two minutes to discuss what went right, what went wrong, and what needs to be improved. Leaders should always support these debriefings and encourage providers to speak up about mistakes so that the team can learn from them.

• Create the 5 filters. This involves having regular discussions with all team members—nurses, front desk staff, physicians, laboratory staff, and technologists—about the things that put the organization at risk. Within these conversations, teams should discuss the following:

—What are the 5 diseases that put our patients at risk (such as asthma, diabetes, depression)?

—What 5 medications put our patients at risk (Coumadin, insulin, and so forth)?

—What 5 abnormal test results should we watch out for (such as an abnormal biopsy or abnormal EKG)?

—What 5 diagnoses can we not afford to miss (such as a heart attack in the clinic)?

This discussion gives all staff members a heads-up on patients' risks, so they are looking for high-risk patterns. What is very valuable is the dialogue among the team members as they learn and evolve the filters. From these discussions organizations should create checklists and processes of what to look for/what to do regarding these filters. For example, an organization may create a checklist for Coumadin use that can be followed whenever a patient is put on Coumadin. You choose 5 filters, because that is a manageable number that staff members can wrap their head around. If you ask staff members to watch out for 35 different critical things, they will not be able to reliably keep track of any one thing, and the process will become ineffective.

• Address patient health literacy. As discussed in Chapter 9, it is important to provide education materials in a format patients—all patients both literate and illiterate—can understand. While staff should be aware of the signs of low health literacy, providing a standard of care in which all patients are educated using easy-to-understand materials and in which education is confirmed using repeat-back and teach-back methods, is critical to ensuring patient safety. The Joint Commission requires organizations to engage in such culturally competent care.

• Develop a systematic process for responding to critical test results. As part of the 5 filters discussion you should define the short list of critical test results. After that is defined you should be clear what the information pathway is and who owns the responsibility to inform the patient and act on the results. Through NPSG.02.03.01, The Joint Commission requires organizations to measure, assess, and, if needed, take action to improve the timeliness of reporting and the timeliness of receipt of critical tests, and critical results and values by the responsible licensed caregiver.

• Develop a systematic process for following patients who go into the hospital and managing the transition from primary care to the inpatient arena and back.

• Develop a reliable process for coordinating care for patients who see multiple providers. It is critical in ambulatory care to have some central repository for patient information. This helps ensure that all the providers of care—the primary care physicians, hospitalists, and specialists—are kept up to speed on the patient, care decisions about the patient, and treatment outcomes. On a very basic level, this helps prevent the patient from being on medications that negatively interact and cause harm.

CONCLUSION

Throughout this publication, we describe the process of cultural change, performance improvement, and reliability as a journey, and yet it is a journey that never really ends. It is not a one-time event or a six-month process. Achieving safe and reliable care requires continuous action. A decision to pursue such care is a commitment that requires organizationwide participation and constant vigilance. It must be a basic property of the culture, where the goal is doing the right thing for the patient every time.

REFERENCES

1. DeFontes J., Surbida S.: Preoperative safety briefing project. *Permanente Journal,* 8:21–27, Spring 2004.

2. Carthey J., et al.: Behavioural markers of surgical excellence. *Saf Sci* 41:409–413, 2003.

3. de Leval M.R., et al.: Human factors and cardiac surgery: A multicenter study. *J Thorac Cardiovas Surg.* 119:661–672, 2000.

4. Edmondson A.C., Bohmer R., Pisano G.P.: Speeding up team learning. *Harvard Business Review,* Oct. 1, 2001.

5. Uhlig P.N., et al.: System innovation: Concord Hospital. *Jt Comm J Qual Improv* 28:12, Dec. 2002.

6. Uhlig P.N., et al.: The John M. Eisenberg Patient Safety Awards. System Innovation: Concord Hospital. *Jt Comm J Qual Improv* 28:666–672, Dec. 2002.

7. Pronovost P.J., Sexton J.B.: Assessing safety culture: Guidelines and recommendations. *Qual Saf Health Care* 14:231–233, 2005.

8. Jha A.K., et al.: Patients' perceptions of hospital care in the United States. *New Engl J Med* 359:1921–1931, Oct. 30, 2008.

9. Hayes C., et al.: Retaining oncology nurses: Strategies for today's nurse leaders. *Oncology Nursing Forum* 32, Nov. 2005.

10. Bosk C.L.: *Forgive and Remember: Managing Medical Failure.* Chicago: niversity of Chicago Press, 1979.

11. Makary M.A., et al.: Operating room briefings: Working on the same page. *Jt Comm J Qual Patient Saf* 32:351–355, Jun. 2006.

12. Mazzocco K., et al.: Surgical team behaviors and patient outcomes. *Am J Surg,* Sep. 11, 2008.

13. Human factors and cardiac surgery: A multicenter study. *J Thorac Cardiovasc Surg* 119:661–672, Apr. 2000.

14. Leonard M., Frankel A., Simmonds T.: *Achieving Safe and Reliable Healthcare.* Chicago: Health Administration Press, 2004.

15. Pronovost P.J., et al.: Implementing and validating a comprehensive unit-based safety program. *J Pat Safety* 1:33–40, 2005.

16. Joint Commission Resources: *Managing Performance Measurement Data in Health Care,* 2nd ed. Oakbrook Terrace, Illinois: The Joint Commission, 2008.

17. Resar R., et al.: Using a bundle approach to improve ventilator care processes and reduce ventilator-associated pneumonia. *Jt Comm J Qual Patient Saf* 31:243–248, 2005.

18. Pronovost P.J., et al.: An intervention to decrease catheter-related bloodstream infections in the ICU. *N Engl J Med* 355, Dec. 28, 2006.

19. Bellomo R., et al.: A prospective before-and-after trial of a medical emergency team. *Med J Australia Rapid Online* pp.1–5, Aug. 18, 2003.

20. Whittington J., et al.: Using an automated risk assessment report to identify patients at risk for clinical deterioration. *Jt Comm J Qual Patient Saf* 33:569–574, 2007.

21. Joint Commission Resources: *Best Practices in Medical Emergency Teams.* Oakbrook Terrace, Illinois: The Joint Commission, 2006.

Appendix

A Systematic Approach for Reading Fetal Heart Tracings

Michael Fox

As discussed in Chapter 13, Michael Fox and colleagues from the University of California, San Francisco created a systemized approach to monitoring and interpreting fetal heart tracings. Fox's approach suggests the risk specific fetal heart rate (FHR) patterns have for the development of a significant acidosis in the fetus can presumptively be predicted based on the degree of baseline FHR variability that accompanies the pattern.[1-3] This suggests that three general categories of FHR patterns can be identified:

1. FHR Patterns Not Associated with Significant Acidemia—the presence of **moderate variability.** An FHR tracing with recurrent decelerations of any type and/or second-stage bradycardia, when accompanied by moderate variability, 6–25 beats per minute (bpm), **is strongly predictive of the absence of significant acidemia and the presence of neonatal vigor at birth.** This is a good clinical situation to be in.

2. FHR tracing with **minimal variability, in association with recurrent decelerations of any type and/or second stage bradycardia, is associated with significant acidemia and the absence of fetal vigor at birth,** but the consistency of this association is uncertain.

3. Patterns Inconsistently Associated with Significant FHR Patterns Associated with Significant Acidemia— **absent variability in association with recurrent late decelerations, variable decelerations and/or a sustained bradycardia of ≤ 60 bpm, are the FHR patterns most consistently associated with significant acidemia and the absence of fetal vigor at birth.**

A Systematic Interpretive Construct:

1. **Look the baseline FHR variability first.** Why?

Because FHR decelerations as an independent finding are poorly predictive of complicated outcomes. Instead the degree of baseline variability that accompanies the decelerations is the most sensitive indicator of the adequacy of oxygen delivery to the fetus at any given moment. Importantly, the presence of moderate variability is evidence the fetus is adequately oxygenated, at that moment, whether or not the moderate variability is accompanied by recurrent decelerations or second stage bradycardia. Conversely, absent and/or minimal FHR variability, accompanied by recurrent decelerations and/or a sustained bradycardia of ≤ 60 bpm, are the FHR patterns most consistently associated with a significant acidosis in the fetus.

2. **Look for the presence or absence of recurrent fetal heart rate decelerations and/or bradycardia.** With the exception of acute catastrophic events, metabolic acidosis typically develops in the fetus slowly, in association with recurrent decelerations and an evolutionary reduction of FHR variability over time. In addition, there is a positive relationship between the degree of acidemia and the depth of the decelerations. In the setting of recurrent decelerations or sustained bradycardia the magnitude of the decrease in the FHR appears directly linked to the rapidity with which acidemia may develop.

3. **Monitor the baseline fetal heart rate.** Traditionally, the baseline FHR has been identified and communicated first, yet it is rarely of principle importance unless it is extremely high (tachycardia > 200 bpm) or significantly low (≤ 80 bpm remote from term, ≤ 60 bpm at any time). Again the significance of the baseline FHR is more accurately determined based on the degree of variability present at the time of its assessment.

4. **Examine the evolution of the tracing.** The ability to

Figure A-1. Fetal Heart Rate Tracing

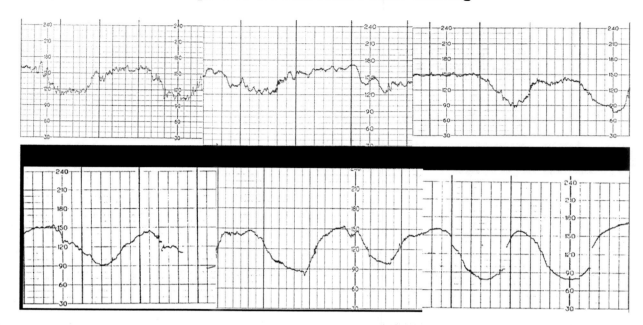

This figure demonstrates the evolution of an FHR tracing as it loses its baseline FHR variability in association with recurrent decelerations. In Box 1 (upper left), we know there is a 99% chance the fetus is adequately oxygenated at that point. By the time we get to the lower right, Box 6, we have an unacceptably high chance that the fetus is being compromised. If we have a tracing that is evolving with a loss of variability and recurrent decelerations, we want to deliver the child in a timely manner.

Source: Tracing courtesy of Michael Fox. Used with permission.

appreciate pattern evolution and to recognize and understand changes in the FHR tracing over time is the key element of FHR interpretation. Studies support the premise that FHR variability will become diminished or absent before significant fetal acidemia develops. As a general rule, during the intrapartum period a hypoxia-induced reduction in FHR variability develops gradually (commonly over 60–120 minutes), and occurs in the context of minimal or absent variability in association with recurrent late, variable, or prolonged decelerations (*see* Figure A-1, above).

Providers can improve the accuracy, choice, and timing of their interventions by first determining the evolution of the tracings, based on the degree to which the tracing exhibits more variability, less variability, or remains unchanged from previous time periods. This emphasis on pattern evolution reinforces the importance of observing the tracing for evolutionary changes in the FHR variability, particularly when recurrent decelerations or bradycardia are present. Put simply, is the tracing going in the right direction or wrong direction? If the tracing is losing variability in

association with recurrent decelerations the bedside providers then must determine who needs to be aware of the situation. Who needs to be at the bedside and how quickly? And when to intervene?

ADDRESSING EMERGENT FHR PATTERNS

Rapid delivery of a fetus in a safe and timely fashion should be a routine accomplishment for any obstetrical service. Most discussion of emergent cesarean section has focused on "decision to incision time." Studies of the effect of "decision to incision" times on ultimate neonatal outcome have failed to conclusively establish a benefit in the 30-minute guideline.

The Event to Delivery Interval

Studies of obstetrics cases resulting in significant morbidity/ mortality suggest the "event to delivery" interval is of critical importance. This period begins when FHR changes associated with presumed fetal acidemia first present on the tracing or are appreciated through auscultation. The bedside provider must recognize the variant FHR pattern; make a presumptive assessment of the fetal status; notify the primary provider; and accurately communicate his or her findings. The primary provider must determine the significance of the tracing or auscultated patterns and initiate appropriate management. Management options range from the initiation of conservative measures that are aimed at abolishing the variant pattern, institution of continuous monitoring, C.N.M./M.D. consultation, development of a plan for collaborative management, or, in cases of presumed fetal acidemia, transfer of care and preparation for immediate operative/surgical delivery. The selection and timing of interventions should be consistent with the patient's condition, and additionally take into account geographic constraints (travel time from home to hospital of M.D., C.N.M., anesthesia, operating room (OR) crew, pediatrician), institutional and national guidelines, and other logistic factors.

THE 3 Rs OF EMERGENT DELIVERY

Given the complexity associated with emergent delivery it is important for the OB team to have a simple and consistent response to emergent situations. When an FHR tracing becomes acutely complicated a host of traditional nursing and medical interventions are generally employed. These commonly include position change, fluid bolus, hyper-oxygenation, discontinuation of Pitocin, Terbutaline administration, and scalp stimulation, to name a few. If used randomly, these routine measures, may delay the implementation of more important and central maneuvers. At the core of a timely and effective response to presumed fetal jeopardy is the assessment of three key clinical variables, which can be remembered by the pneumonic RATE, ROUTE, ROOM. In rapid sequence:

- RATE: The FHR tracing is evaluated to determine if an emergent response is truly warranted or if conservative measures and continued observation are appropriate (variant pattern vs. presumed acidemia). If the inciting event is iatrogenic (maternal hypotension from epidural administration, tetanic contraction from Pitocin, etc.) treating the presumed cause of the inciting event will usually result in a rapid resolution.

- ROUTE: If the fetal heart rate pattern suggests emergent delivery (a diagnosis based on the severity of the pattern, lack of response to conservative treatment, addi-

tional clinical variables), a sterile vaginal exam should immediately be performed, unless contraindicated, to assess whether the fetus can be delivered vaginally or if a cesarean section is required.

- ROOM: Based on the assessment of the fetal heart rate and the information derived from the sterile vaginal exam, it should be determined whether vaginal delivery is imminent and help and equipment should be brought to the patient or whether it is more appropriate to move the patient to the OR for assisted or surgical intervention.

The 1-2-3 Guideline

There are no clinical studies that suggest an absolute time frame before conservative measures (position change, fluid bolus, hyper-oxygenation, terbutaline administration, etc.) should be abandoned and the patient moved to the OR for emergent delivery. Outcomes from a large series of uterine ruptures indicate a window of opportunity between *12–17 minutes* is generally available depending on the status of the tracing and fetus prior to onset of the bradycardia.

Providers must simply be mindful of the protective benefit of delivering the fetus with a bradycardia within this window of 12–17 minutes. Keep in mind that too much time spent in a labor room employing conservative measures may result in an unwarranted delay in accomplishing the ultimate "cure"—delivery.

In the middle of the time pressure, chaos, and sense of danger that accompanies bradycardia, a simple way to think about when to move to the OR is to remember the 1-2-3 Guideline.

During the **first minute** of a deceleration ≤ 60 bpm the bedside provider can observe the tracing for evidence the pattern is resolving, attempt to correct the source of the problem, and do a sterile vaginal exam, and clearly communicate the results of such. This will quickly establish for everyone involved the likely route of delivery, if it should be necessary.

By the start of the **second minute** additional help should be mobilized, and the room be made ready for easy exit in the event the pattern does not resolve.

By **minute 3** move to the OR unless you have a good reason not to do so. Pragmatic considerations simply suggest when a fetal bradycardia of 60 bpm or less does not resolve to quickly move the patient to the OR and be prepared for delivery. Once in the OR, "resuscitative" measures can be continued while the patient is prepared for delivery. Clear, simple rules in stressful, high-risk situations deliver great value. These two simple algorithms; RATE, ROUTE, ROOM and 1-2-3 help providers to predetermine relative priorities, and improve the accuracy and timing of critical interventions.

Consider the following example. The nurse at the bedside sees a prolonged deceleration of fetal bradycardia that does not recover—the heart rate drops from 140 per minute to 60. This baby is clearly in trouble. A large series of uterine ruptures from USC–LA County shows that with an acute interruption of blood flow, if the baby is delivered within 12–17 minutes, there is a 99% chance of a successful outcome. This is a situation that requires a timely and consistent response. In the RATE, ROUTE, ROOM model, the nurse has 1 minute to try to fix the problem—supplemental oxygen, positional change, etc.; by minute 2 she has a colleague present trying to help; and by minute 3 they have done a sterile vaginal exam, recruited help, and are physically moving to where this child is going to be delivered. This is not a situation in which the team wants to waste time in the room if an emergent C-section is needed. The clock is running. Move the patient to where the problem can be solved in a timely manner. What's the worst thing that happens here? The patient gets better and they go back down the hall. Compared to a possible bad outcome, we'll take that every time.

The advantage of this system is twofold. It pushes commonality in the interpretation of relevant clinical information and reinforces a consistent response to the information received. To help facilitate the fast response, organizations should have a designated code in which activation prompts an automatic page to all relevant providers, including physicians, anesthesiologists, nurses, and so forth. In an emergency, one page should bring everyone you need running. Having to page six different people and wait for them to call back invites mistakes and wastes time. A pager that shows CODE PINK 911 is a pretty clear message that says "run, don't walk."

REFERENCES

1. Fox M., et al.: Fetal heart rate monitoring: Interpretation and collaborative management. *J Midwifery and Women's Health* 45, Nov. 2000.
2. Boehm F.H.: FHR variability: Key to fetal well-being. *Contemporary OB/GYN* 9:57–68, 1997.
3. Parer J.T., et al.: Fetal acidemia and electronic fetal heart rate patterns: Is there evidence of an association? *J Matern Fetal Neonatal Med* 19:289–294, 2006.

Index

Q

R

S

T

U

V

W